D0776849

SECOND OPINION

SECOND OPINION

The Columbia Presbyterian
Guide to Surgery

Eric A. Rose, M.D.

A Lark Production

ST. MARTIN'S PRESS
New York

Book design by Susan Hood

Library of Congress Cataloging-in-Publication Data

Rose, Eric A.
    Second opinion: the Columbia Presbyterian guide to surgery/ Eric Rose.
        p.   cm.
    ISBN 0-312-20584-8
    1. Surgery—Decision making.   2. Surgery, Unnecessary—Prevention.
3. Patient education. I. Title.

RD27.8 .R67 2000
617—dc21

99-089285

First Edition: March 2000

10   9   8   7   6   5   4   3   2   1

A Note to the Reader

Acknowledgments

This book, like virtually all surgery, is the product of extensive collaboration. Special thanks to Joanne Kabak for her skill with words. Deborah Schwarz-McGregor, P.A., and Robin Dellabough were the driving forces behind translating a concept into a manuscript. The narrative chapters in Parts One and Two were inspired by the questions of patients and their families, as well as the seemingly endless queries of medical students and residents. It is just these simple issues that shed the most light on what we know, and, equally important, what we need to learn and communicate. The operation-specific chapters in Part Three were primarily the work of Columbia Presbyterian surgeons, whose expertise and diligence in responding to "simple" questions reflect their remarkable commitment to keeping patients well informed as an integral part of the process of getting well. They are listed in the resource section.

In addition, there were many Columbia Presbyterian staff members and other professionals who provided invaluable information beyond the scope of specific surgical procedures. Their knowledge informs the entire book. They include Suzanne Arcuni, orthopedic surgery; Dr. Ellise Delphin, anesthesiology; Dr. Beth Ann Ditkoff, breast cancer surgery; Dr. Andrew Feit, anesthesiology; Dr. Seth Feltheimer, internal medicine; Michelle Gabay, RN, surgical oncology; Tom Hickey, P.A., cardiothoracic surgery; Dr. Paul

LoGerfo, thyroid surgery; Wahida Karmally, MSRD, director of nutrition; Anne B. Lawler, CSW, social worker, heart failure and pretransplant center; Dr. Mehmet C. Oz, cardiac surgery; Ellen Simon, Ph.D., Director of Social Work; Dr. Joseph Tenenbaum, cardiology; Sandra Walsh, director of patient relations; Diana Walsh, administrator, thyroid; Jery Whitworth, director of Department of Complementary Medicine; Grace Wong, medical insurance.

—*Eric A. Rose, M.D.*

Contents

Contents

Contents

Introduction

You might assume that I, as chief of surgery at a major medical center, would be in favor of surgery. So why do I think the world needs a book called *Second Opinion*? The story of two octogenarians I saw in one recent week will help explain.

They both came to me for heart bypass surgery. One was a very sick eighty-three-year-old. This man was taking every medicine available, including many nitroglycerin tablets daily. He was in constant pain. A heart bypass operation held substantial risks for him. So, in light of his advanced age, I asked if his pain was so bad that he was willing to risk a 20 percent chance of dying to be rid of it. His answer was, "Hell, no. I'll live with it. I don't want to go through an operation. I'd rather live with this pain, understanding that I may even die from it in the next few days."

The same week, an eighty-six-year-old came in. This man swam one hundred laps a day, but he was experiencing angina at the fiftieth lap. He said, "I've had a rich and enjoyable life, and swimming is very important to me. I'm willing to take the 20 percent chance of dying to be able to swim without pain." After a successful operation, he's swimming 100 laps a day again.

The first patient chose to live with his pain. The other patient wanted to get rid of it entirely. Both of them made a reasonable choice, but the point is that it was *their* choice—not the doctor's decision.

Most people at some time will have to face whether they or a loved one should have an operation. The consequences of that decision are enormous. Everyone has the potential ability to evaluate and participate in the decision. No matter what your condition, you do have certain choices, in terms of *what* operation you may need, *where* you're going to have it, and *whether* you're going to have it. You need to make those choices using the best knowledge you can obtain so that you get the best outcome: to feel better and live longer.

I wrote this book to provide you with the information you need to make informed decisions concerning surgery. This is truly a *self-help* book. Although opting for surgery is a way people can help themselves, many people have a remarkable lack of insight into the process. I want this book to empower you to take charge of your own care with the surgeon as your collaborator. You can and should play a key role in the decision-making process.

I tell my patients if they're uncomfortable with what they're hearing from me, they ought to get a second opinion. Don't have surgery because you like the way the doctor's office looks, or because he's a friend of a friend. Instead, you should be convinced of two things:

1. You understand what your medical problem is.
2. You understand how an operation is going to help you solve the problem.

There are several major themes in the book to help you think about surgery in the most logical way. Part One covers the basic question: "What's wrong?"—not always as simple as it sounds—and addresses how surgery may solve whatever is wrong, along with its benefits and risks. The big question is: "What are the problems I am trying to solve?" You can't figure out what to do until you really narrow down what's wrong. Is your problem *I don't like my eyelid wrinkles* or *I've got coronary disease?*

You begin to take charge of your health by asking your doctor to explain what it is he or she thinks is your problem. It doesn't have to include the gruesome details, but rather an understandable description in lay terms. For example, a doctor might summarize your condition by saying, "You have stones in your gallbladder that are causing inflammation which, in turn, is causing you pain. This is called cholecystitis." Or, "You've torn the ligaments in your knee, which means that your knee is unstable and will hurt if you exert yourself."

The second thing any patient needs to understand is the proposed solution, and its benefits and risks. Part One of this book addresses the general questions you can ask no matter what kind of surgery is involved: *"Why is this surgery going to help me?" "How?" "What are the downsides?" "Can this surgery hurt me?"*

The answer to the last question is almost always yes. So the real concern is, how *likely* is it that the surgery will hurt you? Sometimes there is simply not enough quantitative data to answer all the questions, but you certainly should be able to get a good sense of risk versus benefit.

Risk is intrinsic to all surgery, starting with the ultimate risk of death. You could say that almost any procedure has *some* death risk. I urge patients to put this particular risk into perspective. Walking across the street has *some* death risk. In surgery, infection, bleeding, and complications of anesthesia are the most common risks.

Taking these risks into consideration, you next need to find out exactly what benefits the surgery would provide. For example:

- It will stabilize your knee, allowing you to play tennis with less pain.

- It will make your eyelids look like you're twenty-three years old.

- It will keep you from having a heart attack.

- It will eliminate your gallstone pain, or has an 80 percent chance of eliminating your gallstone pain, leaving you with a 10 percent chance of still having a little pain, and a 10 percent chance of still having as much pain as you had.

The biggest mistake people make is to have surgery for the wrong reasons. Ask yourself, "Is this surgery going to make my life either longer or better?" If you can't answer at least one of those questions in the affirmative, you shouldn't have the operation.

Obviously, if a doctor is telling you that because of your problem you may be dead in a week, you can't ignore such a warning. Yet surgery isn't always as urgent as a surgeon makes it seem. Unfortunately, there are some physicians who pressure patients with questionable results. For example, a woman who has chronic back pain sees an orthopedist or a neurosurgeon. She hasn't asked all the questions as to what the alternatives are, or things haven't been explained sufficiently to her. She has the recommended operation, and four months later, she still has back pain. She's back to square one. After having taken considerable risk, she wonders why there hasn't been any benefit.

I can't emphasize enough the importance of a patient taking responsibility for his own health. Sometimes a patient is so frightened by the prospect of surgery that he can't think about it. Surgeons have a term for an inability to consider one's own choices: *autonomy dumping*. It places a big burden on the physician, who has to be highly ethical in pointing out to the patient that he is essentially giving up his autonomy. It's better to *want* to understand your own surgery, which should be explainable. If the physician can't explain the surgery in plain English, you should be highly suspicious.

Consider, too, the fact that there are several alternatives to surgery. First is simply to accept the problem, to do nothing. Second is to use conventional medical therapy, such as medication, exercise, and rehabilitation, if it's available for the problem. Many people are under the impression that surgery and other therapies are mutually exclusive. They think, "If I have angina, I'm either going to have an operation *or* I'm going to have medical therapy." These procedures are not mutually exclusive. They can often be used to complement one another.

Depending on the problem, simply waiting is definitely another alternative, often the best. For example, roughly 85 to 90 percent of back pain disappears on its own with the passage of time. Let's say you sprain your back. If you see a neurosurgeon who immediately orders an MRI, CT scan, and a spinal tap, it's probably an unnecessarily aggressive response.

Another myth I hope this book dispels is that choosing surgery will solve the entire problem in one fell swoop. In fact, operations are generally not curative. They're most effective when combined with ongoing strong medical management. For example, you smoke, are diabetic, and have a high cholesterol level. Then you have a small stroke. You may be able to prevent future strokes by having an operation called a carotid endarterectomy. However, the surgery alone is *not* a cure-all. It's a big help and improves the prognosis. But if you really want the full warranty for the operation, you need to stop smoking, get your cholesterol level down, and keep your diabetes well controlled. A good surgeon will advise you of this.

After you've read about the process of deciding to move ahead with an operation, Part Two discusses the logistical details: everything you need to do, ask, and know after you decide to have an operation. *"What time do I show up in the hospital?" "What medicine should or shouldn't I take?" "Are there any consultations I should have beforehand?" "Do I see the anesthesiologist?" "Would seeing a hypnotherapist to help with relaxation techniques be a good idea?"* The more you know about the procedure ahead of time, the better prepared you will be for the recovery period.

Part Three covers the nuts and bolts of forty-five of the most common surgical procedures. Each procedure is described precisely and clearly with illustrations to further aid your comprehension. Not only are the basic steps of the operation clearly explained, but presurgical testing that may be needed, potential complications, and post-operative recovery are also addressed. This section will be invaluable in explaining to concerned family, friends, or post-operative care providers exactly what is happening to your body in surgery.

All any patient wants to hear is that his problem is solvable, or manageable, and that he is in competent hands. The single most reassuring thing that I can say to a patient is, "I think I can help you." If you're contemplating any kind of surgery, I think I can help you.

Part One

———

DO I NEED
SURGERY?

1

Understanding Your
Medical Problem,
and Its Surgical Solution

No one ever wakes up one day and says, "Gee, I'd really love to have an operation." Everyone wants to feel better, look better, live longer, and stay disease-free, but no one wants to be cut open, endure discomfort, and put normal activities on hold.

Yet it's a prospect that faces millions of people each year. Surgery is not inevitable, but it is quite likely that you or someone you care about will someday have to consider it as an option.

How you do react when surgery is recommended? With a sense of relief that there's help for your problem? Or with a denial that you even have a problem? Are you hit by an overwhelming desire to have the operation right now? Or do you just go numb, letting the doctor's words float out of your consciousness?

There are as many ways to react as there are types of surgery. No matter how you first react, try to make the effort and take the time to find out why an operation is recommended, what it entails, and how your health will improve.

If you decide to have surgery, it should be for a very specific reason: you are convinced that it is the medical alternative that supports your best interest.

It helps to recognize a point that can get buried in the emotions aroused by the word *surgery*. When you hear your diagnosis, you are not just a patient in a doctor's office—you are also a consumer buying a very important service.

3

It may seem a strange concept at first, especially for those who grew up in an era when the doctor gave the orders and the patient did as told—no questions, no options. But it isn't crass to question your doctor. Nor does it imply disrespect to professionals who have studied and practiced for years. If you are concerned about offending your doctor, remember this: doctors *expect* you to ask lots of questions, perhaps get a second opinion, and possibly end up following a different strategy than the one they originally recommended.

You can compare the situation to any major purchase. The stakes are very different, but wouldn't you expect to put at least as much effort and ask as many questions about an operation that could alter your life as you would about buying a car?

You want the medical system to work to your advantage. After all, you are buying into a treatment package—physicians and staff, medical center, type of operation, recovery plan—that will make a difference in the quality, even the length, of your life.

I urge you to establish from the outset that you have a big role to play. *Be proactive.* You can break your responsibilities down into these ten steps:

1. Choose medical professionals who are caring and knowledgeable.

2. Gather the facts of your medical condition through testing and discussion.

3. Obtain a clear description of your diagnosis and treatment alternatives.

4. Put that description into the context of what it means for your everyday life.

5. Create a support team of friends and relatives.

6. Confirm your diagnosis and treatment options through a second opinion.

7. Evaluate the risks and the benefits of your options.

8. Understand what happens to you during the operation, in recovery, and post-operatively.

9. Form realistic expectations of what an operation can accomplish.

10. Decide whether or not to have surgery.

Of course, if there is a medical emergency and your life—or the way you live it—is in immediate jeopardy, you may have to have surgery on the spot without going through this sequence. When there *is* a choice, however, try to use these steps to help you make the *best* choice.

Taking the time may be tough, given the risks of surgery, the expense, the immediate impact on your lifestyle, the demands it places on your family, and the rigors of the recovery process. But it is worth every ounce of effort you put into being a proactive consumer in the surgical process. Understood and used properly, surgery can provide powerful benefits for you.

In some cases, the decision is fairly easy to make. You're clear about what you want and the medical data confirms your best option. In others, the decision will take a lot of probing, discussing, and researching to answer the question: *"Do I need this operation?"*

Surgery can be daunting, but it need not be shrouded in mystery. It is a process that includes finding out what's wrong and repairing it. It's common to get stuck on images of the operation itself in which you appear as an unconscious body on an operating table while the surgical team—gloved, gowned, and masked—uses a formidable array of instruments on you.

No wonder people anticipate an operation with concern, if not terror. What an ultimate act of trust! You see yourself as giving up all control to a surgeon who is going to have to subject you to trauma without question. In return, you expect to gain better health and a longer life. It is an agreement that no reasonable person enters into lightly.

Your participation in the decision-making process of surgery can lead you to enter into that agreement wisely. You exercise control beforehand so you can feel safe in the operating room. But your role in treating your medical condition doesn't mean you have to operate! You are not expected to pass the scalpel, advise the surgeon, or monitor equipment during the operation. That would be absurd.

But it is also unthinkable, unless you are in an emergency,

that you would end up in an operation without knowing who is operating on you, why you're there, and what benefits will result from it.

Your intention to get the best information possible and your belief that the decision is yours to make will lead you to a realistic goal: to have the data in your hand and the feeling in your gut that having that particular surgery performed by that specific surgeon is the best option for you. Being wheeled through the operating room doors is not the beginning of surgery; it is the culmination of the process.

Collaborate or abdicate?

Just because a procedure is doable doesn't mean it should be done on you. Your best approach is to view the process from the start as a collaboration between you and your doctor, not as a predetermined course from which you cannot veer. You and your physician need to listen to each other to understand what is relevant to create an outcome that best suits your needs.

What, then, can you bring to the discussion? Doesn't the doctor, with his experience, data, and presence of mind hold all the cards?

No. *You* have the critical pieces that complete the puzzle of how to proceed:

• What is important to you?

• Can the result of surgery make *your* life better?

Even in a medical crisis, the answers to these questions are an indicator of whether the solution to your problem is surgery, alternative treatments, or doing nothing at all. The level of medical intervention should be a reflection of what fits the way you want to live your life.

For example, perhaps you have a condition called claudication, which is debilitating pain in your leg(s) when you walk due to blockages in the arteries of your leg(s). The choices of treatment range from medication and exercise to placing balloons and stents in the arteries to an operation to bypass them. How do you choose?

You'd start by thinking about your lifestyle in the context of the medical problem at hand. If your favorite activity is running six miles a day and you've had to give that up because of the pain, the level of treatment you seek is more likely to be at the high end of the spectrum than if you are a couch potato who rarely walks more than a block at a time.

The many other questions you'd ask, including whether you could lose the limb in an extreme case, are more meaningful if you see the interrelationship of your lifestyle with your treatment options.

If physicians were treating only the disease process, their job would be a lot easier. But they are treating the whole person and they need to know your thoughts and concerns to map out a plan with you. When one person hears that a lump that's been discovered in his thyroid is benign, he may be so relieved he's ready to fly out of the office. Another person may be so fearful of having any lump at all, that he could only live happily if he has it removed.

It is not responsible for the surgeon to follow a treatment course simply because you, the patient, want it, if he thinks you can be harmed by it. Nor is it his job to predict what you want; it is your job to tell him as clearly as you can.

A breast surgeon determined that the cancer in a young woman could be successfully treated by the standard method of removing the lump *and* the lymph nodes along with radiation. However, the woman insisted she only wanted the lump removed, nothing else. Rather than do an operation he considered substandard, the surgeon referred the woman to a radiologist and an oncologist so she could find out more about the impact of making that choice.

Of course, you can also opt out of this whole process and let the doctor decide. You can say, "I don't want to hear anymore. I'm too upset about this. Just go ahead. I trust whatever you want to do." Such autonomy dumping, as I've mentioned, is an option. It's quick and easy. But most people, when they consider the consequence of handing over a decision that could have a major impact on their lives, think better of it. At the very least they may say, "I trust what you're going to do. Tell me about how you'll do it and what the outcome will be."

In some cases the patient is mentally impaired, too young, or too old to make the decision for himself. You may be called upon to go through all the steps of the decision-making process for this loved one. The question remains the same: given the set of facts and the lifestyle needs of the person who is depending on you, is surgery in his best interest?

In answering the question of whether or not to have surgery, you may find that the process of collaboration by its very nature leads to some disagreements. Feel free to speak up—as well as to be challenged in turn. It's the give and take that leads to clarity, different perspectives, and finally a consensus. As long as you and your physician treat each other with mutual respect and are open to new insights, you're on the right track.

How do I begin?

You should not be daunted by the prospect of learning about disease and surgical repair. Like all big efforts, you start with small steps. You do not need to know every nuance, every last detail. You do not need to acquire the same level of knowledge as the physician. What you do need is to get the information that will allow you to feel comfortable about making a decision.

"Doctor, what's wrong with me?"

It may happen that you arrive at the doctor's office for routine tests or an evaluation of symptoms. And you leave with a recommendation for surgery. You should expect to get the following information from the doctor with whom you're consulting:

- An opportunity to describe your symptoms, ask your questions, and express your concerns.

- An understandable, coherent explanation of the disease or injury you have.

- A description of its specific implications for you and for your quality of life.

You need to hear your physician describe, in plain English, the basics of your medical condition. If it helps you understand better, ask for pictures and diagrams along with a verbal explanation.

As one woman who had surgery put it, "If I ask the questions, I get the answers."

Imagine discovering you have a heart condition called aortic stenosis. An ideal dialogue between you and your doctor would be the following:

What is aortic stenosis? It's an abnormality of the aortic valve that guards the left ventricle. The valve is located at the spot where blood leaves the major pumping chamber of the heart.

What does that valve do? When the valve is normal, it lets blood flow freely out of the heart and keeps blood from leaking back into it.

What's wrong with my valve? It's gotten so narrow that it's difficult to eject blood from the heart and to prevent blood from leaking back into the heart.

How do I experience this? You could have shortness of breath, chest pains, or fainting episodes. Or you may have no symptoms.

Adapted to your condition, these questions are your opening salvo for understanding any medical problem and deciding how to treat it. In more general terms, this is what you're really asking:

- What part of my body is diseased or injured?

- What does it do when it's operating normally?

- What's it doing in my case?

- How does this affect me?

How can I tell if I've had enough tests for an accurate diagnosis—or if I'm having too many tests?

There are many types of tests for most medical conditions. The question to ask your doctor is: "Will the information obtained from this test help us make a meaningful decision about my problem?" If not, then the test is not necessary.

A doctor feels comfortable with the thoroughness of the testing process when he has enough information to establish a definitive diagnosis and to exclude reasonable alternative conditions.

When your doctor provides his diagnosis and explains how he reached it in a way that makes sense to you, you can be assured that the testing process was thorough and complete.

Given my medical condition, what will surgery do for me?

There are two main reasons for recommending surgery:

- To prevent death or a catastrophic illness.

- To relieve symptoms.

It may sound simplistic but remember, no operation will make you feel better if you aren't suffering from symptoms. If your heart valve isn't working properly, but you don't have shortness of breath or chest pain, you won't experience improvement in how you *feel* after the operation. What you *will* experience is the knowledge that you've substantially reduced your chance of dying from a heart attack in the near future.

If you're having an operation to keep from getting worse (e.g., preventing the spread of cancer or a heart attack), the questions to ask are: What's the likelihood of preventing death or serious illness if you have the operation or if you don't?

If you do have symptoms, know which ones you're addressing, which will remain, and which will go away. Sometimes people who undergo surgery have a vague sense that an operation will fix a lot of things that are bothering them, although they're unrelated to the specific surgery. If you have chest pain *and* leg pain, you can expect to eliminate the discomfort in your chest from valve surgery. It will *not* eliminate the pain in your leg!

Find this out before the operation. You don't want to go into an operation with unrealistic expectations about what is going to change, only to come through it disappointed.

Most decision-making about operations today is based on data from observations of large populations over long periods of time, expressed statistically. Even if you're the type of person who shunned statistics in high school math, try not to block it out when it pertains to surgery. You need to combine an understanding of the scientific data on surgery with your own personal medical history.

You'll undoubtedly hear stories from friends and relatives about how Uncle Joe had the same operation, and did—or did not—benefit from it. Sure, you'll be tempted to get emotional reinforcement from anecdotal evidence. It may be your only personal exposure to that type of surgery to date. And most people are only too willing to share their war stories. But don't get hung up on anecdotes.

These stories are intriguing but are no more than a rough guide to what is going on with you. Medical treatment is a highly individualized process. You are unique and that uniqueness determines which option is best; furthermore, methods and techniques may well have changed since the time of your relative's surgery.

How do I look at risk in deciding whether I should have surgery?

Assessing your tolerance for risk is a concept that's often applied to activities like investing your money, but it's also entirely relevant in a surgical context. Risk permeates the surgical process, including how likely it is you will improve through surgery. For example, if you have back pain and there is a chance that it will recur after surgery, you would want to know if that chance is 2 percent or 30 percent before you decide on the operation.

Looking at the numbers helps you put your medical condition in context of what is *likely* to happen to you, not what is *definitely* going to happen. One woman in her mid-forties found out she had colon cancer and a section of her colon was removed. Although she had surgery, her doctor said that in the future she still had twice the chance of getting cancer in another part of her body and ten times the chance of getting colon cancer again than the average person.

Ten years later, when tests showed some abnormal-looking cells in her colon, she was faced with a decision of whether to have surgery to remove them. The doctor said he felt 95 percent sure that the cells should be taken out. She went ahead and had the surgery. No cancer was found. The statistics helped her decide on the need for the surgery; they were not a guarantee of the outcome. She didn't feel her surgery was unnecessary. Given her risk factors, she felt it was a wise decision. Her overwhelming sense was one of relief that all was well.

You place confidence in your physician's ability to identify the statistics that have a direct bearing on the surgery you're considering, and to make them understandable. You want to know answers to questions such as:

- What are the chances of curing the problem through surgery?

- What is the chance that specific symptoms will improve?

- How much improvement can I expect in how I feel or in my life expectancy?

- What is the chance the symptoms or disease will recur?

- Where do these figures come from and how valid are they?

What are the risks associated with the surgery itself?

The type and level of risks vary widely, depending on the operation and your medical condition.

Fear is a normal response to these risks, but you can find out whether that specific fear is irrational or not. Ask yourself, "What am I really afraid of if I have an operation?" Once you pinpoint your fears, you can express them to your surgeon. Do not feel embarrassed. Many people are afraid of anesthesia or pain. Others fear being out of work or having a scar. Doctors have heard them all and would much prefer to discuss your fears than allow them to prevent you from having surgery or to make you miserable.

Risks of surgery include:

Mortality. Yes, you can die in surgery. The risk ranges from virtually 0 to 50 percent and up. Highly invasive surgery creates a greater likelihood of something happening that could threaten your life. In an operation to replace a heart valve, the risk of dying in surgery is about 2 percent. In an operation for breast cancer where the surgery is basically on the body's surface and there is very low chance of bleeding and infection, there is much less risk.

As a result of going through an operation, you could suffer a heart attack or stroke, have bleeding, get an infection or pneumonia, have kidney or liver failure. But the chance in your case may be so minimal that it's not a factor in your decision. With another set of medical facts, the risks may have to be weighed more.

Concerns about mortality are real, but there is a way to deal with them: bring them out into the open. Allow yourself to get relief from knowing the facts. You may stay up nights worrying about anesthesia and when you finally decide to speak up, the doctor says, "Don't worry about it. There's a greater likelihood of being killed in a car accident on the highway." That might help you put your fear into perspective: why obsess over anesthesia when every day you drive to work on the highway without feeling any undue fear that this is the end?

Pain. The amount of pain you may experience is totally variable and depends on the operation. You can't assume how much pain there will be based on the type of operation. In the aftermath of some types of heart surgery, there is less pain than after an operation for a dislocated shoulder. If you're concerned about pain and how to relieve it, speak up. Don't go into surgery dreading pain or worrying that you sound weak if you insist on having appropriate measures to relieve it.

There are many strategies today for pain relief. The spectrum of drugs is remarkable and continuing to grow. New techniques have made it possible for some patients to control the administration of drugs for their pain. Ask your doctor to discuss whether you are a candidate for pain relief without drugs, including self-hypnosis, physical therapy, deep-breathing techniques, and massage.

Everyone has a different threshold of pain and a different way of reacting to it. One person has a headache and keeps on functioning; another takes medication and goes to bed. How one experiences pain is an individual response, so don't try to compare yourself to some mystical "normal" pain threshold. Rather, be aware of how you react to pain and expect appropriate relief from *your* experience of it.

Fatigue. This is a universal complication of surgery. Studies have shown that any one of the components of surgery—anesthesia, bed rest, lack of food—can bring on fatigue. When you put them all together, it's no surprise you're knocked out.

Even in minimally invasive surgery, recovery can take a long time. In many cases, your medical condition debilitates you to begin with, which will, in all likelihood, delay your rate of recovery after surgery.

Often patients feel okay in the direct aftermath of surgery, only to feel worse in about three days. Then they gradually start to improve. If you know this in advance, you can understand the recovery phenomenon and not be afraid that something is wrong when normal post-surgical fatigue sets in.

Other complications from surgery include: infection; bleeding; stroke; heart attack; allergic reaction, nausea, and vomiting from anesthesia; and reopening of the wound. Your surgeon should discuss all the risks frankly with you. Find out what may cause a problem during or after surgery and whether it applies to your situation. As a quick reference, read about a specific surgical procedure in Part Three of this book, page 161–313.

In evaluating whether to have surgery, consider what's worse for you—the risks associated with surgery or those associated with a disease or injury left untreated?

In theory, it sounds great to ask all these questions, but I also imagine a waiting room full of patients. How can I expect the doctor to spend the time with me?

Most physicians today are very busy people. They have to respond to time pressures, life and death emergencies, *and* your questions. You can't carry on a collaboration without respect for a doctor's time and demands.

Nor should you be so bowled over by the doctor's pace that you feel like you're being bulldozed out of the office. Don't be intimidated and fail to get the answers you need; *be proactive.* Stop the doctor in his tracks if he seems to be rushing you out the door. Clearly state that you feel pressured and need to ask more questions. If it's impossible for him to talk further at that moment, ask, "What time can I call you so that we can continue this discussion?"

Your primary relationship is with your physician, but he is not the sole resource for the information you need. In a well-run practice, there is a highly skilled support staff to cover all your concerns and questions. They include:

- *A physician's assistant or associate (PA).* A PA is a licensed, certified clinician who works under the supervision of a physician. If the doctor has a PA in his practice, it is very likely he will participate in your treatment and be a significant resource for your questions. PAs go through an abbreviated medical school program that typically lasts two to three years. They take classes and do hospital rotations alongside medical students. Some go on for further training in a specialty like surgery.

14

- *A nurse practitioner (NP)* is a registered nurse (RN) who has advanced education, such as a master's degree, and extensive clinical experience. Under regulations that vary by state, a nurse practitioner is generally allowed to work alone or with a medical team and to examine, diagnose, and prescribe medication for patients. Nurse practitioners work in primary care and in a number of specialties, for which they may be certified by a national board.

- *Explanatory materials.* These brochures are available through the doctor's office. They are produced by organizations like the American Cancer Society; hospital publications and videos; newspapers and magazine articles from the lay press; and journals from scientific organizations.

- *Hospital services.* Volunteers who have had the same disease are often available to talk to you on a one-on-one basis, and support groups are some of the resources that hospitals can provide.

- *Web sites.* Some sites are very useful, including those from hospitals and medical organizations. But you have to proceed with caution as to the validity of other health sites. Anyone can apply for a URL and set up a Web site, so be aware that the content of such sites may not be accurate. (Note: There is a resource list of reliable Web sites on page 319.)

The upshot of the information-gathering process is that you feel your questions and concerns have been answered. Similarly, the surgeon is also gathering more data through additional tests and consultation with colleagues. Deciding on a course of action can take one visit, or several.

But what if I get the sense that I'm *bothering* the doctor if I come back with more questions or ask to hear something over again?

If you are not comfortable enough with the responses from the physician and staff you are consulting with, you have a couple of options.

One is to confront the physician with your feeling that your concerns are being rebuffed. Most will respond to that. You can press the doctor in a direct and firm way. "So, you are telling me my only surgical option is a mastectomy? What if I refuse to have a mastectomy? What other options are available to me?"

Of course a doctor can be a skilled surgeon, yet may have difficulty talking to his patients. Or he may be a world-renowned specialist with time restrictions even greater than the average doctor's. In those cases, your concerns still should not be ignored. You can say, "I am not happy with how unavailable you are for my questions but I don't want to switch doctors. Can we work out a way I can get my questions answered?" The doctor should understand your need to know more and connect you to a medical professional on his staff who is qualified to answer all your questions in his stead.

If you still don't think the doctor is being responsive enough, you can go to another doctor. Consider whether you want to put yourself in the hands of a person who can't communicate adequately with you, and who, when you express your concerns, still resists giving you appropriate information about your condition.

How am I going to remember all the information I'm getting?

Estimates show that within twenty-four hours, about 75 percent of what a doctor discusses with a patient is usually lost. Without a doubt, there is a great deal you have to absorb and consider. You may be feeling ill or anxious, and in any case, hearing the risks of disease and surgery are not part of your normal routine.

There are several ways to overcome that loss of information. Remember what works for you when learning something challenging. What would you do in your job, for example, when you're taking on a new task? You can apply the same techniques here.

- *Simply listen.* For some people, that's all it takes.

- *Repetition.* The first discussion you have with a physician is not likely to be your last. He expects to repeat information to you; you will also hear the information again from staff, such as the PA. And you can read about the topic in the materials you've gathered. Redundancy here is not a waste of time; it reinforces your learning.

- *Bring someone with you.* A friend or a family member can help you remember and discuss what was said. It is an invaluable asset to have a "lay consultant" with you when you visit the doctor. Since your companion is not personally on the line in the same way you are, he is likely to hear the information more clearly.

- *Take notes.* If you're comfortable doing so, bring a pen and paper and write down key points during your visit.

- *Tape the discussion.* You can play it back in the quiet of your home later, as well as share the information directly with family members. Some doctors also make a tape, especially when they are confirming your informed consent to a procedure. You can ask for a copy of that tape.

How do I choose who to bring with me?

In tracking your illness and recovery, one of the important choices to make is the selection of your personal support staff. Who do you trust to bring to doctor's visits? With whom can you really discuss your personal feelings and medical data? Who will be objective? There are no absolutes—even in the basic matters of who goes with you and with whom you discuss your medical concerns. You are in charge of how you move forward, and lining up your team is part of controlling how well the process flows.

The options vary here. Your major consultant, like a spouse or a parent, may or may not be the best person to bring with you to an office visit. If someone is anxious, and will only feel more so in a situation such as this, you might absorb that discomfort. The tension could affect your ability to concentrate. You may want to review the information with that person at a calmer time later in the day. Bring another relative or a friend instead, someone who can sit and have a cup of coffee after the appointment or who has the ability to make you laugh even in the tensest moments.

Someone in your family might feel bad because he's been left out of the information loop regarding your treatment. Or another person may not want the responsibility of helping you make this decision, and may say no to your request to go visit the doctor with you. The whole process is very stressful for the family members involved, who are also coping with your illness. As a person dealing with a medical challenge, you may not want to deal with the reactions of family, including feelings of rejection. This is a time to center on yourself, so you may have to explain to others that you are making the choices that work best for you at this moment.

Surgery is a major life occurrence, and as such, it does provoke reactions in relationships. And it's not always reassuring. In some cases, such as for an elderly person, the input of relatives is very important. But family members can have their own agendas. Many a doctor has consulted with relatives, especially where a will may be involved, only to be asked a little too eagerly, "He's going to die—isn't he?"

Concerned relatives really can make a positive difference. When an elderly woman was diagnosed with breast cancer, her doctor told her to have a lumpectomy and radiation. Her relatives were concerned. Why didn't the doctor tell her also to have the lymph nodes removed, a standard procedure to see if the cancer has spread? Was it because she was older and he figured it didn't matter as much for her? In fact, the woman loved life and wanted to do everything possible to prolong it. Her relatives took her to another surgeon where they discussed all the options in a standard treatment program.

Sometimes relatives serve as translators passing along information. "Dad, what the doctor is telling you is. . . ." And sometimes they see themselves as gatekeepers, holding back information. If dad's brother recently died of a stroke, they may decide it will make him too anxious if he hears that there is a small risk of stroke during the operation. On the other hand, what if dad gets an infection after the operation that requires another surgery and he's never been told it's a possibility? A patient can get very upset if he finds out information was being withheld only to have a problem he never expected.

Ideally, the patient should be informed fully, since he's the one going through the operation, but doctors will also respect the family's input on this matter. A doctor is unlikely to say to the family, "I don't care what you think, I'm going to tell him anyway." At the very least, the doctor will make sure someone in the family has a complete grasp of what could happen.

The operating principle here is who, and what, is in the *individ-*

ual's best interest, whether you're picking a physician or a treatment plan, and whether it's for you or for a person you're helping.

In the following pages, we will take a closer look at just how you can find the right surgeon and how you can make the best choices of treatment through getting a second opinion and gaining an understanding of all your alternatives.

2

Getting a Second Opinion

When an eighty-year-old woman in Florida developed shortness of breath, she went to her doctor to find out what was wrong and what could be done to alleviate her symptoms. Her cardiologist ordered diagnostic tests that confirmed a leaky heart valve. His recommendation for treatment was immediate surgery.

"Not so fast," said the woman's daughter when she found out her mother had already checked into the hospital. "Why the rush? What are the alternatives?"

The daughter insisted on a second opinion. She sent her mother's records to a cardiologist in New York and got another evaluation by phone. Medication was not only an appropriate alternative to surgery, the second cardiologist said, but given this woman's needs and condition, it was the best choice.

In an ideal world, the doctor will describe the pros and cons of all reasonable treatments for your condition. But as in the case just given, it doesn't always happen. Even when you are fully versed in all of the treatments available, you still may not be sure which one to pick.

How can you confirm or challenge a diagnosis and treatment plan when this may be the first time you have heard of the condition? You can't expect to have a command of medical detail or the broad perspective that comes from years of training and experience. But you can speak to someone who does. It's called getting a second opinion.

Come to think of it, when have you ever relied on a single source when you've made a major decision? When you buy a car, you probably spend a string of Saturdays at dealerships, talk to other car owners, pore over consumer evaluations, and read up on gas mileage and repair records.

As a consumer of medical care you should do no less. You don't have to fumble around, trying to figure out how to get another opinion. There's a system in place that doctors are quite familiar with: they look at the data in your particular situation and give you an opinion on it even though you're not their patient. It's an intelligent way to get at least one more answer to a compelling question: "What is best for me?"

Do I *have* to get a second opinion?

No. It's your choice. Some people feel secure enough about what the first doctor has told them that they feel they don't need to get more input.

For one fifty-year-old woman who had severe pain in her knee from a fall on the ice, one opinion suited her just fine. She went to her family doctor who recommended an orthopedic surgeon; not only did her doctor know the surgeon's work professionally, but he also knew his work personally. The surgeon had operated on the family doctor's wife, with good results. When the woman consulted with the surgeon, she felt comfortable with their conversation and confident in his skills.

First the surgeon recommended physical therapy. When that didn't work, he recommended surgery on her knee. She didn't feel the need to speak with another physician on the matter. She went ahead with the operation, and the pain improved dramatically.

In another case, a man in his forties injured his back and went to see a neurologist who diagnosed mild sciatica and recommended physical therapy. The pain worsened so much that the man couldn't work. It seemed to him that the neurologist was too low-key about his problem and so he pressed for further testing.

In response, the neurologist scheduled a diagnostic test called an MRI. But the testing location the doctor chose was more than an hour from the patient's home. The appointment was at night, when driving was very difficult for him. Nevertheless, he went to the appointment. As he drove, he realized that the doctor's insensitivity had been demonstrated yet again. After the man endured the inconvenience and discomfort of the drive, he found out the same test could have been scheduled much closer to home. All this only deepened the sense of concern he had been feeling about the doctor. He decided to send the results of his test to another specialist for a second opinion.

The first neurologist read the results and said there wasn't a big problem. The second neurologist said he had a ruptured disc that required surgery very quickly. The patient got an appointment with a top spinal surgeon and had the operation within days. The pain went away. He went back to work and, eventually, to running and competing in triathlons!

Two patients with pain, two treatments that started out with physical therapy and ended with operations. Yet one person had good results with a single opinion; the other needed a second doctor to get well.

There is no magic formula to follow. In deciding whether to go for a second opinion, ask yourself the following kinds of questions:

- How serious is my condition?

- Should I be getting independent verification about the information I've heard?

- Is there any chance that I could be following a course that's not the best?

- How big an impact will the decisions I'm making now have on my life?

- How do I feel about my doctor and my interaction with him?

- Do I have any doubts about anything I've heard?

- What do I have to lose if I take my records across town and say to another doctor, "What do you think?"

For example, for most women with breast cancer there is a choice between saving the breast and removing it entirely. But not every physician describes that choice adequately. A second opinion may be the only way some women realize that they have options.

Sometimes, people with a diagnosis like cancer are so angry that they believe the doctor can't possibly be right. They have high expectations that a second opinion will refute the first diagnosis. Even if that hope isn't fulfilled, a second opinion can go a long way in emphasizing the reality of an illness and in shedding light on the different methods of treatment.

The idea of doing even the minimal research that a second opinion entails is just too alien for some people. They make decisions, like buying stocks, on the recommendation of a single person they know and trust. And that's how they're going to invest in their medical care.

Recognize where you are on the spectrum of personality types and medical situations. But don't be ruled by simple inertia. If all signs point to a second opinion as being in your best interest, why ignore them just because you can't be bothered?

Are there any circumstances when I should clearly get a second opinion?

A second opinion is particularly important for a person who is considering a nonstandard treatment or experimental procedure.

For example, a new type of surgery, called sentinel lymphadenectomy, to see whether breast cancer has spread by removing only the first lymph node under the arm, rather than all the lymph nodes, is currently being evaluated. The procedure is far less demanding and painful for the patient during surgery and in its aftermath. It may be standard within a couple of years for those with early breast cancer; as of this writing, it is not.

If a patient is presented with this procedure as an option, she needs to understand that long-term results aren't known yet. The removal of just the first node may prove to be insufficient to detect the spread of cancer. Until it is proven that this new procedure works, it must be explained to patients why the standard procedure is still being done. However, there may be circumstances under which the experimental procedure alone is a viable option.

But in the highly competitive field that medicine has become, some physicians may be suggesting removal of just the first node as though it was a standard rather than an experimental treatment. Is the patient being given the information she needs to make a decision? Does she fully understand the risks and benefits? This is a case when a patient would clearly benefit from having a second pair of expert eyes to look over the treatment plan. Discussing the procedure with another physician may bring to light any misconceptions relating to the treatment approach.

At what point should I get a second opinion?

Sometimes people look for another opinion right after they get the initial one. They don't leave the doctor's office without at least one recommendation for a second opinion. For others, the decision to get an independent appraisal comes later.

You don't want to go in search of a second opinion the day before the operation, if you can help it. A second opinion is not a last-minute attempt to deal with panic about an impending operation.

Nor does it make sense to drag out the process. You may well feel that the nature of your problem and the state of the available treatments make it necessary not only to get a second opinion, but even a third, or more. At some point, you recognize that you have enough information to make an informed choice. Otherwise, you should question whether you are getting additional opinions as a way to postpone what may be an inevitable need to have surgery.

What happens if there's an emergency?

Don't hold up your treatment in order to get a second opinion when you are in a life-threatening emergency or where the risk of harm from delaying a procedure outweighs the benefit of taking another look.

Say a patient has chest pain that is so persistent and recurrent that it does not respond to medical therapy, even to powerful drugs given intravenously. When a device, called a balloon pump, is inserted, it too barely controls the pain. The individual needs coronary bypass surgery very quickly. The physician recognizes that to wait longer is completely unacceptable. There may be time to explain that to the patient, but there isn't time to spend a couple of days getting another opinion.

If a patient is adamant about getting a second opinion, the doctor should make sure that the patient understands what the impact of waiting might be, including how much it increases the chances of having a heart attack or dying. In some cases, there may be time for a relative to talk to another doctor on the phone, but the conversation will need to be brief.

How do I know if I have time to get a second opinion?

Ask the question directly: "Is there urgency? What would be the consequences of my exploring this option for a few hours? A few days? A few weeks?"

In general, if symptoms are stable, there usually is time to consider the various choices. But it can also happen that a patient comes in for diagnostic tests and evaluation, finds out there is a serious illness, and feels compelled to stay in the hospital and have a procedure done right away. The sense of urgency becomes so great that the patient doesn't even go home first.

Sometimes it's an institutional push—from a business point of view, you are a bird in hand. Sometimes the urgency is accelerated by a patient's fear. Try to calm down and find out if you are in imminent danger. If you aren't, then take the time to evaluate your illness and treatment. Do not be railroaded into making a major decision or just give up under the stress of the diagnosis. Typically, there are several weeks or longer after a diagnosis in which a person can evaluate his options.

But what if I know my doctor well? Am I not insulting him or her by saying I want another opinion?

Not at all. It is standard medical practice to get another opinion. Doctors do it all the time as part of their own process of diagnosing a problem. You should not feel any qualms or guilt about stating that you want a second opinion. Many physicians will give their patients the names of other specialists and surgeons to talk to without even being asked.

One of the beauties of our medical system is that you can make decisions among various options. But sometimes people mix up their priorities. Ironically, a person can take it for granted that he can go to a supermarket and choose whatever he wants. However, that same person, when dealing with a health issue of major importance, somehow feels he doesn't have a right to make a choice. Rather than tell his physician he wants to talk to another doctor, he'll fall silent. Imagining that he might hurt his doctor's feelings if he gets another opinion, the patient just does what he's been told.

Any physician who makes a patient feel uncomfortable about seeking a second opinion is doing that patient a major disservice. Keep in mind it is your body, your life, and you have the right to do everything you feel is necessary for your health.

How do I find a second opinion?

Methods of obtaining a recommendation for a doctor who will give you an opinion include the following:

- *Ask your physician.* Doctors generally know who's skilled, has a good reputation, is the best in the field—and who's not. You may have to go no further than your primary-care physician, specialist, or surgeon with whom you're consulting to get the names to call for your second opinion.

- *Talk to family and friends.* As with any recommendation, you turn to people you trust and who have some knowledge of the subject. If a friend has gone through an operation, he'll likely give you his honest appraisal of the surgeon. You still may want to get more information from other sources, but tapping into your own network of word-of-mouth references is a reasonable place to start compiling a list of physicians to contact.

- *Call hospitals, medical societies, and organizations.* Many have 800 numbers and physician-referral services. This is a more impersonal approach than getting a recommendation from your doctor or your brother. Yet it does allow you to access a database that identifies physicians within the specialty you are seeking who practice in your area. Similarly, Web sites are also a resource for names of doctors. (See Appendix A, Resources, on pages 314–20.)

- *Contact your insurance company.* Since you want to be reimbursed for your consultation, in most circumstances you will be consulting with a physician who is part of your plan. Beyond simply getting a list of names, find out if your insurance company is also a resource from which to get more information or specific recommendations about the physicians who are enrolled.

What if someone refers me to a doctor who practices in the same medical center as the original doctor?

Keep in mind an independent appraisal means a different doctor, but it doesn't have to be a different institution. You should realistically expect that a doctor from the same hospital will give an honest, objective opinion on your medical choices even if it challenges the opinion of a colleague.

Is it better to go outside your original doctor's medical center? There is no easy answer to this question. One way to look at it is to consider what makes you feel comfortable. You should not be surprised if the doctor who is treating you gives you the names of other physicians at the same hospital for your second opinion. If you aren't happy going that route, you can ask your doctor for names at a different hospital or use one of the other aforementioned options to get references.

How do I process all this information?

By now, you probably realize that little in the process of finding out what is best for you is a matter of simply accepting what you're told. You want your second opinion to be an important link in the chain of information that leads you to a wise choice. Just because you have a name and phone number of a doctor who is a specialist in your area doesn't mean your task of finding a second opinion is over. You need to consider carefully whether you have found someone whose skills will be an important factor in confirming or challenging your treatment options.

Weigh the names you've collected, asking yourself questions like:

- Is my insurance company referring me to a practitioner who is best at evaluating surgery, or best at controlling costs?

- Is my friend referring me to his cousin because of his reputation, or because he needs to build up a practice?

- Is the hospital I'm calling a distinguished academic or community institution, or have I never heard of it before?

All this research may be hard to handle if you're not feeling well or are upset by the diagnosis and its treatment options. This is a good time for you to call on your personal support team of family and friends to do some of the legwork and confirm the validity of references you've received.

Who is going to pay for a second opinion?

As with all matters relating to medical coverage, you have to call your insurance company or the human-resources or benefits department where you work and find out what your particular plan will cover and what it will not. In the past, insurance companies often required a second opinion for surgery. This is less common now.

It is reasonable to think that if you choose to have a second opinion, your insurance will pay for it, but you have to make sure. If you have questions about how to approach your insurance company, ask for help from the staff at your doctor's office. They are likely to have experience in what you need to provide. The benefits department of your employer will also act as an intermediary between you and the insurance company.

What if you want to consult with a physician who is not covered within your insurance plan? Say he does an uncommon procedure that you are interested in finding out about. For example, there is a thyroid surgeon who performs a type of biopsy that few others do. He can point to statistics that show he is able to eliminate a lot of unnecessary surgery since this type of biopsy is more precise in identifying what is malignant and what isn't. Unfortunately, the surgeon is not currently participating in any managed-care plans.

You have a couple of choices if you find yourself in a situation like this. You can appeal to your insurance company before making an appointment. You can file a claim with them after the visit with the reasons why you believe they should pay it. Or you can decide to pay the doctor's bill yourself. A consultation would cost about $200. Is this an amount you are willing or able to pay to get an opinion about your medical condition?

What am I looking for in a second opinion?

You generally want an appraisal of the diagnosis you've been given and of the treatment that's been proposed for it. Be very direct in telling the second doctor that this is what you are after. "Here is what my doctor told me about my condition. He recommends surgery. What do you think?"

The process is similar to getting your first opinion. The physician reviews the facts, explains the illness, discusses the treatment options with their risks and benefits, and answers your questions and concerns.

When you go for a second opinion you are already more knowledgeable than when you first were told of your medical situation. You have heard a diagnosis, asked questions of your physician and his staff, read relevant material, and discussed the options with people you trust. You probably have zeroed in on the questions about which you are most concerned.

This time, you have the results from your original consultation, which you should bring with you to your appointment. Sometimes, the second physician wants more information, including additional tests. It is up to you if you want to do them, and where. If you've traveled a distance to get the second opinion, you may prefer to go back for additional testing closer to home. As long as the information is reliable, it is reasonable to go to a place that is convenient for you.

Will I get an opinion on the spot?

If the physician has all the pertinent facts, you should expect to get a frank opinion quickly.

Will the doctor make the decision for you? No.

It is okay, however, to ask a physician to step outside the role of the medical professional and say how he would feel if he had to make the choice for himself or his family. The closest you can come to having the doctor fill in for you is to ask him to answer the following question: "If you were me now, if you had the particular set of problems that I'm experiencing, would you go ahead and have this operation?" You are entitled to an answer. But to get the full benefit of this information, you need to ask not just what he would do, but *why* he would do it.

Perhaps the doctor tells you he'd have the surgery because it would make a big difference in his lifestyle since he travels a lot. Maybe you also travel frequently and that helps you see the benefit. If medication is an option instead of surgery, the physician may say he often forgets to take medication and that alternative doesn't work well for him. And you recognize "that's not me" because you're very reliable when it comes to taking your pills. The ultimate decision is yours. The input from the physician can help you frame your decision; he can't make it for you.

I have two opinions from reliable doctors about how to treat my medical condition. Maybe the advice is the same and maybe it isn't. How do I evaluate one in light of the other?

If there is a disagreement, try to understand the reason for the difference of opinion. Specifically go through the arguments for and against each approach. Evaluate the pros and cons yourself, follow up with your doctors, and discuss the matter with a friend or relative who is a reliable sounding board for you. Consider the specific options and the credentials of the physicians giving them to you.

Ultimately, go with your gut. Which doctor do you trust, which approach makes sense to you? If those answers point you in a direction, it probably is the right one.

If neither approach feels right, then go back to your original question. What is the outcome you want? Is it really achievable? If you want to have a nose job, but you aren't satisfied with the opinions you're getting, maybe the issue isn't the surgical technique but the end result. If what you want is Sharon Stone's face, then having a nose job might not accomplish that.

What if you are convinced the outcome you want is achievable? After having two opinions, there is generally lots of information on the table. However, if you feel you still don't have enough information to make an informed decision, then get a third opinion. It's not that commonly done, but it certainly is an option. If you do seek a third opinion, go back to the fundamentals of the medical condition at hand and frankly address your concerns to this third physician.

You can ask the doctors with whom you've consulted to confer with each other—and that you be present. Particularly if there is a disagreement, you may well want to hear the discussion between them. This is an opportunity to air the differences and see if an open discussion changes anyone's mind.

You do not have to go through the process on your own of evaluating the merits of conflicting medical opinions. There are fine points that may be well beyond your grasp. And take heart—experience shows that out of the process a consensus generally emerges.

After you've reviewed your first opinion with a second, or even a third opinion, then you've got to create the definitive opinion—yours.

Does getting another opinion always involve going to another specialist or surgeon in the same field?

There are other ways to get helpful input that aren't technically second opinions, including getting a revised opinion from your original physician. You can go back to him with questions on information you've learned and ask, "In light of this, do you still think the course of treatment we discussed is the best one to follow?"

Another is to get an "alternative" opinion by consulting with another medical professional who is not a specialist in the area of your illness. This may give you a fresh perspective on your problem or lead to a useful referral.

It's been more than forty years since one mother had a seriously ill child, but she still vividly remembers how talking about the diagnosis to her gynecologist led to a reevaluation of her child's condition.

Her baby had been diagnosed with an intestinal disorder by a pediatrician. As time passed, the child did not seem to improve. She decided to bring up her concerns during her own gynecological exam. Since the gynecologist had seen the baby at birth, she reasoned, he might have some insight into the problem.

He did indeed. He said the first diagnosis sounded way off the mark and urged her to get another opinion quickly. In a second opinion, the mother found out her baby had a food allergy and not an intestinal disease. Once the child went on a totally different diet, her symptoms disappeared.

Whether it's mother's intuition, a nagging doubt, or a major illness that allows no room for a mistaken course of action, the urge to get another opinion is one to be heeded.

Years after her child's illness, this woman said her ongoing commitment to making the time and taking the trouble to get a second opinion has continued to pay off for her and her family. When her brother-in-law called recently to say he was going to have major surgery to treat an aneurysm near his waist, her response was, "Are you sure? Have you seen someone else?" She finally got him to seek a second opinion, where he learned that because of his heart condition, he could suffer serious harm, even death, in the type of surgery he was considering. After he got that news, he opted for medication instead.

Fortunately, you don't need to accept what you're hearing from a single medical authority. You can easily gain information through another informed opinion, and that can go a long way toward confirming your choice or encouraging you to reconsider.

To make that informed choice, you need to know what your alternatives are, including what's new or experimental. These topics are addressed in the next chapter.

3

Evaluating the Alternatives

The most personal and routine moments of daily life can be directly affected by your choice of treatment for a medical condition. A physician can, and should, lay out all the alternatives, but only you know what is and is not acceptable for you.

For example, two men with an obstructed bladder had to choose between medication and surgery to fix the obstruction. The main symptom of their disease, called benign prostatic hypertrophy, is difficulty emptying the bladder. This usually results in a slow urinary stream and frequent urination. And, although painless, it means waking up a lot at night and being unable to do activities like sitting through a movie without the need to urinate.

Unless your bladder is completely obstructed and you can't urinate at all, the condition isn't life-threatening. It can be treated by medication, which will decrease but not eliminate the symptoms, or by surgery, which removes the obstruction. One man didn't want to have surgery and felt he could live with the symptoms as long as they weren't too hard to manage. For him, medicine was a reasonable alternative. The other man wanted no part of getting up two or three times a night or leaving a performance to go to the bathroom. He chose surgery.

You have to look at the beginning of your treatment with the endpoint in mind. If, for example, you're retired and therefore don't have to arise at a very early hour, then maybe you'd take medication since a few trips to the john in the middle of the night isn't a big deal for you. But what if you're a businessman who frequently attends long meetings? You might find it uncomfortable and embarrassing to excuse yourself several times to go to the bathroom. In that case, the benefit of saving face at the office outweighs the hassle of having surgery.

An option is just that—a choice. Look at it with the sharp eye of a seasoned consumer. Do you need the treatment and want it? Is the "price" you have to pay too high? Will it work for you?

Don't approach your choice like a first-time computer buyer at the mercy of the experts; rather, think of yourself as acting like a discriminating shopper strolling through an ancient bazaar, one who takes the time to smell the goods and finger the cloth.

PERSONAL BELIEFS

When you choose medical treatment, of course it is not the same thing as buying an expensive piece of merchandise. Nor are the issues solely ones that are based on what's technically available, what your insurance policy will pay for, or what approach fits with your business commitments.

Rather, the choice of how to deal with disease and treatment, for many people, springs in large part from their personal, ethical, religious, and spiritual beliefs. You don't just bring your wallet and your appointment book to an important life decision like medical care. You bring all of the components of your character.

For some, specific tenets of their religion affect whether they have a surgical procedure and how. For example, circumcision is an important ritual for people who practice Judaism. Surgery on a Jehovah's Witness has to be performed in the context of that religion's prohibition against the use of other people's blood to keep a sick person alive.

Patients will say to their doctor, yes, they understand everything about the treatment and its likely result, but ultimately they believe the outcome is in God's hands. Deep spirituality can include the belief that what really counts is not what's taking place between a person and her doctor, but what's already been determined between her and the spiritual being in whom she believes. It's not that such people are disinterested in the circumstance of treating their illness, but that they have a profound feeling that the key questions have been dealt with on a different level.

The motivating factor for choosing a treatment is often the value a person places on existence itself. In life-and-death circumstances, some will always choose the option that has the greatest chance of extending life, even if that life comes with misery and suffering. Others put a greater stock on the quality of life and so will reject courses of action they feel will result in a life that, under their criteria, is not worth living.

Many believe that healing comes from within, and they will include prayer, meditation, or other healing rituals along with standard medical procedure to treat their medical problem.

For others, the issues are less spiritual and more physical. Their standards revolve around concerns about how they look or will be perceived by others. Some people reject surgery if they fear a scar will be too ugly or too visible. On the other hand, another patient with disfiguring facial and neck cancer may undergo many operations because the concern about looks is no match for her desire to live.

The physician is not there to change your essential nature. She is there to use her skills and work within the parameters set up by the technical, financial, and personal possibilities of your life and your medical condition.

DECISION MAKING

This section will help you develop your approach in deciding what to do, identify the pointed questions you need to ask, and define the issues that call for serious consideration, no matter what options are available to treat your condition.

In the most extreme cases, your choice of strategies might come down to only two: have surgery or suffer a condition that may significantly impair your life or even end it.

For example, there are no known therapies other than surgery to repair an acute tear of the ascending aorta. Data shows that without an operation, 75 percent of the patients who have such a rupture will soon die from its effects. Faced with this problem, a person has the option of immediate surgery or facing the next day with no better than a 25 percent chance of surviving it.

Given that choice, it's hard to imagine making a rational decision not to have the surgery. Of course, even here, there are exceptions. A patient may have other serious medical problems that have already so limited her prospects for a long and healthy life that putting herself at risk of dying from a ruptured aorta is not an unacceptable alternative for her.

Not all situations are as compelling as those that involve life and death. Yet understanding any medical alternative involves the same two-step process:

- *The natural course of the disease.* What are its current symptoms? Will they remain in this state? Will the disease get worse and cause further impairment? Will you deteriorate or die from it? Or will the problem improve in time, even without treatment?

- *The path of the disease when it's modified by treatment.* Will treatment cure it? How will each of the alternatives affect the disease and impact on its symptoms?

You won't always end up with an either/or choice. There are often several different paths you can take for a problem, using treatments singly or in combination. You may very well find out that the best alternative involves some combination of the available options, such as surgery plus medication.

You also have to decide what you are willing to tolerate. Can medication control the underlying disease, but cause unacceptable side effects? Will the recovery time from surgery devastate your business?

As you consider how to deal with your illness, you are likely to begin hearing about treatments from many quarters. You'll talk to medical specialists, some of whom may disagree with one another's analysis. You'll also learn of the experiences of friends and read about reports or speculation in newspaper articles and on the Web.

Taking all this information into account, you'll have to learn how to make an informed decision.

One way to decide is to use the method developed by a great surgical educator, Dr. Thomas C. King, who for years taught residents at Columbia Presbyterian. He identified four levels of evidence on which to base medical decisions. Decide where your options fall in his system and ask yourself, "From which level do I prefer to make my decisions?"

1. The first level is simple faith. Someone told you this is the right thing to do and you believe in that person, so you do it.

2. On the second level you not only have faith in the person, but you also believe there is a good reason to make that choice.

3. On the third level you know that there's been some amount of rationally analyzed experience that leads you to believe in that choice.

4. The fourth level is access to a compelling set of data arrived at through a systematic, highly controlled investigation. This is a level that goes well beyond faith.

LEARNING ABOUT ALTERNATIVES

At one end of the spectrum, you have the choice to do nothing. Accept your condition as it is and decide to cope with your current symptoms and those that may arise later. You're not likely to choose this alternative if either the risk of major impairment to your quality of life is high or if there is a risk of dying from the condition. But there are other situations people simply live with. How many are walking around right now with a shoulder that pops out rather than having surgery to keep it from dislocating?

Another alternative to consider is to make lifestyle changes. These changes alone may be enough to reach your goal, or they may well be a necessary adjunct to any medical intervention. For example, how does your diet or other habits contribute to your disease? If you're a smoker and you have blocked arteries in your legs, one of the first things to do is stop smoking. If you've had three heart attacks and a cholesterol level of 400, you can't expect any medical procedure to minimize your future risk if you don't also control dietary fat.

How do I find out what medical solutions are available to treat my problem?

Whatever your condition, you are entitled to know the existing surgical and nonsurgical options, and how they compare.

Ask your physician. A specialist in the disease is usually the best resource.

Do independent research. Read about your illness in books, periodicals, brochures, on the Internet. Talk to people who've had similar problems. Accumulate data that will help you have a more informed discussion with your doctor.

Each condition has its own set of alternative treatments. If you've injured your knee, physical therapy may be an option; for certain types of cancers, it may be radiation therapy. For any type of illness or injury, you want your doctor to tell you:

- What else is being done to treat this condition besides surgery?
- What are the positive points of each method?
- What are the negatives?
- How much will the treatment cost?
- Where will I have the treatment?
- Have there been valid studies on its effectiveness?
- Where can I get more information?

A common alternative for many conditions is pharmaceutical management. If your physician does not bring up the topic, ask her outright:

- Can I take medication instead of having surgery?
- How does medication compare to an operation?
- Are there side effects to medication?

- How long will I have to take medication?

- How much will I have to pay out-of-pocket?

- Could the medication interact with other pills I'm taking?

- Can you tell me about any studies that have been done on treating my condition through medication?

- Is there anything else I should know about the pros and cons of going this route?

After you get answers, consider your reaction to the risks and benefits of medication versus surgery. For someone with coronary artery disease, for example, the best alternative treatment is often medication, but these have side effects such as fatigue and impotency. Are you so relieved there's medication, that you can you cope with its side effects, or would enduring them be much worse than having surgery?

How do I evaluate when to have treatment?
Surgery does not happen in a vacuum. There are many personal issues as well as medical ones that determine how you treat your condition and when. Timing may be crucial as you consider your choices. In some cases, the choice is now or never. In many others, there is an option of "later."

For a woman in her early fifties who owns a catering business, the use of her hands in preparing food is essential. So when she suffered severe pain in one hand from a ganglion (a cyst) in her wrist, she decided to have surgery. Since the recovery time was only two weeks, she was able to arrange her work schedule around the procedure and the relief from pain was worth the disruption.

However, she has also developed arthritis in her thumb. The surgery for that problem is more extensive and would mean she couldn't use her hand for eight weeks. This was an unacceptable amount of time to be away from the demands of her business. Instead, she's taking medication, wearing a splint, and working through the pain. And she's considering whether it's best to sell her business. She wants the operation because the pain from the arthritis limits her lifestyle. For her, the question is not whether to have the operation, but when to have it.

Is one of my choices inpatient versus outpatient surgery?

The choice of being an outpatient or an inpatient is often not the patient's to make. An outpatient has surgery and goes home on the same day; an inpatient stays overnight at the hospital. Most paperwork is done well in advance. On the day of surgery, you go directly to the outpatient surgery area and do a minimal check-in. You cannot have your surgery on an outpatient basis if the procedure is one that the medical community says is too risky or complicated to allow a patient to go home the same day. Your doctor is the best one to tell you that. The choice may be further restricted by the rules of your insurance coverage. For example, hernia repair is almost always done as an outpatient procedure. Unless there's a compelling medical reason, an insurance company is not likely to reimburse you for an overnight stay.

What if you say you definitely do not want to go home the same day as your surgery, but your insurance will only reimburse the hospital for the lesser amount of outpatient coverage? If you do not succeed in reversing that determination, then you would have to face paying the difference out of your own pocket.

Sometimes an operation that's typically done on an inpatient basis could be done as an outpatient. Then you do have a choice to make.

Often a patient's choice is based on what kind of help there is at home. If you don't have anyone to stay with you, if you might be in pain or need other help, then you are likely to opt to stay overnight. It is reasonable to want to be taken care of after surgery. If there isn't anyone to do that for you outside the hospital, and you have the choice, either because insurance will cover it or you can afford to pay for it yourself, then there is no need to rush home. On the other hand, if there aren't unforeseen complications and if you do have someone to help you, recovering in your own bed surrounded by the sights and sounds you enjoy may just be the best way to recover.

An overnight stay may be obligatory because the patient has to be observed after anesthesia, or because of the risk of bleeding, the need for pain control, or the possibility of other complications occurring.

The question of whether you stay overnight and for how long is one of the evolving issues for patients. The answer is governed in part by new technologies that make outpatient surgery possible and by financial considerations that make it desirable.

Removing a gallbladder used to be a seven- to ten-day ordeal with a lot of abdominal pain and gastric dysfunction. Now the new standard treatment using minimal-access surgery means that pain is far less and patients routinely stay for only two or three days.

You need to check not only with your physician but with your insurance company. What will your insurance cover? Managed care typically pushes for outpatient surgery if it's an option or for shorter hospital stays. In the 1980s, for open-heart surgery, a patient used to be admitted two days prior to the surgery and stayed in the hospital ten to fifteen days; now a patient typically does not get reimbursed for even one day prior to surgery. The patient comes in the same day as the operation and stays for only about four to ten days.

When I hear the word "alternative" I also think of herbs, hypnosis, and the like. How do I determine if these are useful methods to treat my problem?

Although some alternative treatments have been used in different parts of the world for centuries, they have generally not been subjected to rigorous testing with the modern research techniques now used to study surgery and drugs. However, use of these treatments is growing substantially in this country. You are likely to find practitioners of different types of alternative medicine in your area and to hear a lot of anecdotal evidence from people who say they've been helped by therapies that are not part of conventional medicine.

If you are interested in exploring whether your medical problem can be treated by one of these methods, consider several questions. Will treatment outside the realm of conventional medicine bring you the outcome you want? Could it cause you harm? On what basis are you building your belief in the treatment—because someone told you about it or because you have access to the data that will confirm or refute its benefits?

Further, alternative does not mean inexpensive. Since most insurance companies cover few, if any, methods of treatment outside conventional medicine, what will the treatment cost you? In the absence of hard data, the risk of pursuing an untested alternative to the exclusion of a conventional medical one is that you may be wasting your money—and valuable time for curing or improving your condition. But it is important to note that, increasingly, alternative therapies such as massage and acupunture are covered when used in conjunction with conventional surgical or medical therapy. The two approaches need not be mutually exclusive.

That's what happened to one patient who decided to try the alternative treatment of chelation therapy instead of having surgery. The patient was trying to combat congestive heart failure due to a blocked aortic valve. In chelation therapy, a substance is administered that removes calcium from the body. Calcium can form in diseased areas like a blocked heart valve and the logic is that by removing calcium, you turn what was a hardened valve into one that's pliable and you unblock it. It's been touted by some as an alternative medical treatment for coronary artery disease. However, the medical community does not support this theory. The best current research shows the only way to unblock the aortic valve is to replace it by surgery.

Although the patient got worse during the six months he was on chelation therapy, once he abandoned it, there was still an option available to have surgery. He did have the valve replaced and his health improved.

If you choose to try an alternative medical treatment in the belief that it will improve your condition, make sure you understand the risks. If it doesn't work, will you suffer harm by delaying the recommended approach? Don't feel uncomfortable about talking openly with your doctor about nontraditional treatments because you think she will be angry or annoyed. She needs your complete picture and you need answers to your questions.

There may not yet be a documented body of evidence you can rely on for an *alternative* to traditional medicine, but there is a growing amount of data that identifies techniques that are *complementary* to surgery and pharmaceuticals. Not an alternative to surgery itself, these techniques can be another way to approach the experience of surgery.

From the first time you experience a symptom or hear a diagnosis right through the challenge of coping with a lifestyle disrupted by surgery and medication, you may experience a stress response.

That response plays havoc with your body, taxing your cardiovascular system, overworking your kidneys, and decreasing your ability to think clearly, among other responses.

Studies are still being done on what has validity and what doesn't in combining the resources of surgery and medication with various relaxation therapies. But could it hurt if you are calmer before, during, and after surgery? If surgery is the best alternative, but you resist it because of fear, instead of rejecting the surgery consider dealing with the fear.

Stress may be particularly high at the time of an operation. Recent research has found that, even under anesthesia, people do indeed absorb and process the sounds of the operating room. There are now audiotapes of tonal music and positive messages, such as "your wound is clean, dry, and free of infection" for use by patients actually undergoing an operation. They not only block out disturbing sounds, but may well create an environment that helps decrease the body's stress response and encourages healing.

Meditation and acupuncture have been researched and been found to reduce stress or relieve pain. Some medical centers are setting up complementary-medicine departments to devise individual programs of mind/body therapies. These include techniques like guided imagery and deep breathing to calm the mind, massage and acupressure to relax the body, and tai chi and yoga to soothe the system.

These treatments aren't for everyone. The idea of being hypnotized or doing yoga postures may just bring about more stress. If your medical center has professionals in complementary medicine, they can help you find what does indeed relax you. You are constantly working in partnership with health professionals in your best interest; exploring complementary-medicine techniques is a way to broaden that partnership.

It feels like there is so much to consider. Isn't it just safest to "go for the gold," and instead of trying to find out about everything else, do the conventional procedure in the standard way?

Not necessarily. Over time the gold standard can become more like tarnished silver. Or tin. This is not the time just to do what you're told or accept what's always been done. The question to ask is whether the standard procedure is still the best, or has a better one been found?

NEW TREATMENTS

If you remember the days when a woman went under general anesthesia for a breast cancer biopsy and woke up without knowing whether she still had a breast, then you can well appreciate the benefits of discovering new methods of treating disease.

The process is a dynamic one. New discoveries, like better ways to treat breast cancer, are being made regularly. What is a standard treatment today may well have been experimental or controversial not long ago. That poses an additional challenge for someone who has to make a decision among treatment options that also include a new procedure still being evaluated. You may be one of the first to have a procedure that thousands will eventually have—or you may be one of the last to have a treatment that'll end up being rejected because it's ineffective or too risky.

You should expect that your doctor will tell you about all the alternative treatments of your illness, including any that are new or experimental. If she doesn't, ask her if recent research has found any new method. Then probe further:

- Does it work?

- Is it safe?

- Could it be better for me than the standard treatment?

It's not just a matter of looking outward, but inward, too. Do you have a high tolerance for risk, a desire to be on the cutting edge? Or do you sleep a lot better at night if you follow the tried and true? Do not feel pressured to choose a treatment because it's new or it's "hot." You have your own comfort level—and you have to live with the results of your choice.

Again, the focus is on achieving an outcome. The surgeon may use a laser instead of a scissor, an electric cautery, or a knife. When there are several ways to accomplish a goal, the ultimate question is not the technique itself, but which tool will get you to the end you want.

When it comes to treatment alternatives, can I assume the latest is the best?

Sometimes the old, reliable standard still works just fine. If a lot of data and experience show a very high chance that you'll get the outcome you want, with little risk, why try something in its place?

In the case of a condition in which a patient suffers from a hole in the heart tissue, there is a new treatment available. The standard treatment was to repair the hole with open-heart surgery. Now there is an alternative of having the hole plugged with a device that's floated to the heart using small catheters going through blood vessels. Among other complications, however, there is a possibility that the device will break off, travel to the brain, and cause a stroke. The amount of data on this procedure is small and cannot yet conclusively demonstrate safety and effectiveness.

The standard operation, on the other hand, is one of the least complicated open-heart operations a surgeon can perform. The chance of the hole reopening after the surgery is basically zero, and there is almost no chance of dying during the surgery itself.

Would you do anything rather than have open-heart surgery? Is there a compelling reason not to have the operation? Are you willing to take on the risks of the new treatment? Or is the deciding factor for you the weight of positive data supporting the standard surgical procedure?

At the other end of the spectrum, a patient may be diagnosed with a disease for which there is no standard therapy that is safe and effective, such as an undifferentiated brain tumor. Here, with everything that's been tried—surgery, radiation, medication—the speed at which this disease progresses is still high and the chance of survival low. If you learn that there's an experimental treatment, one that may cure a condition that to date has been incurable, your response may well be "get me to the cutting edge."

If you're tempted to opt for what's new because you figure what's high-tech has to be an improvement, be sure to get that assumption verified. There can be an entirely different set of risks and unknowns with a new treatment.

There was a time several years ago when the treatment of choice for peptic ulcer disease was gastric freezing with an instrument called a cryoprobe. For a while it was a popular option—until the ulcers came back. No one is freezing ulcers anymore.

Just because someone is touting a high-tech instrument to you now, doesn't mean it will stand the test of time. So when evaluating a new treatment, ask the following questions:

- Is there a standard treatment that reliably produces the outcome I want?

- Will I have enough information to be reasonably sure about the results of the new treatment, or am I part of an experiment?

- How much experience does my doctor have with the new treatment?

EXPERIMENTAL TREATMENTS

At some point, a treatment that's experimental today may be the recommended standard in the future. You need to consider the advice of your physician and your own psychological makeup to decide if you want to participate in a procedure with significant unknown results.

As mentioned in Chapter 2, there is a new procedure, called sentinel lymphadenectomy, to determine whether breast cancer has spread in patients whose cancer is detected very early. Even if there is a low risk that it has spread to other parts of your body, the physician doesn't know this with an acceptable level of certainty until she looks into your body. The standard way to do that has been to remove all the lymph nodes under the patient's arm for examination. In the new treatment that's under evaluation, a surgeon injects a blue dye or radioactive substance around the breast lump and traces it over to the armpit. That leads to the first lymph node, which is the only one removed. It's a much easier surgery for the patient to endure. If that lymph node is negative for cancer, then chances are the rest of the armpit is too, and no other nodes are removed. If the first node is positive, the standard procedure of removing all the rest of the lymph nodes is then followed.

The direction in which the research is going points to a high likelihood that it will become a standard procedure in the near future. However, as of this writing, there is still not enough data to support that opinion.

If you are having breast cancer surgery, your choices today may include:

- *Have no part of the experimental technique.* Do only the standard procedure and have all the nodes removed.

- *Do both.* Have the experimental treatment done along with the standard procedure. You will thereby be participating in the research. Your surgeon will examine the first node in detail and compare it to the others, validating whether the first node gives enough of a basis to judge whether cancer has spread. There is no direct benefit to you as the patient from doing both, other than the fact that the first node is examined more carefully.

- *Be part of a random study and be selected to have either the standard or the experimental treatment done.* When you enroll to do this you don't know which procedure will be done. You will need to sign a special consent form that shows you thoroughly understand what you are agreeing to do.

- *Conclude that you want just the new procedure despite unknowns.* In this case, you accept the risk that cancer is not being detected by the usual means available. You might still prefer this choice now because you trust your surgeon's judgment that it is okay for you to do it. Furthermore, there are immediate benefits. One of the most feared results of lymph node surgery is lymphedema, a painful swelling of the arm. This technique eliminates that complication. The aftermath of the surgery is also less painful, there is no need for drains, and it can be done on an outpatient basis.

In many cases, a consensus does emerge about a new procedure that states the opinion of a reputable medical organization like the

National Institutes of Health. However, that consensus emerges slowly, as experience accumulates and research works its way into publications. That's fine down the road, but what if your personal time frame is now?

It is not easy to be a patient facing the choice of having a procedure that's still in the experimental phases. Both the benefits and risks are often bigger, making the decision tougher. And there is generally a long time during which a given technique falls into a gray zone, where enough testing has been done to show a procedure has merit, but not enough to be convincing that it is better than the standard. Your doctor may tell you frankly, "We don't know which is better."

That gray zone becomes larger when you consider that an established therapy for one person may be an experimental therapy for another. The points in between the poles of acceptable and risky can become so undefined that something truly experimental ends up sounding like standard procedure.

It's not just an individual issue, but a societal one. For example, in deciding when a medical device like a mechanical heart valve can be used as a standard piece of equipment in Europe, the burden of proof for regulatory approval is satisfied when it's shown to be safe. In this country, the Food and Drug Administration (FDA) requires that a device not only be shown to be safe, but also effective.

If you truly believe an experimental treatment may help you or if you have no other alternative, then don't run from a new approach because it's scary to go into relatively uncharted water. Nor should you dive into it lightly, deluded by your own unrealistic expectations or railroaded by an overly enthusiastic doctor.

Enrolling in an experiment is a serious step, one that is guided by established protocols, which should be carefully followed.

First and foremost, understand that you cannot be the subject of an experiment in the United States without agreeing to it by signing a specific informed consent document that identifies the terms of the experiment and demonstrates that you clearly understand what you are doing.

Further, no experiment can be conducted unless it is reviewed and approved by the Institutional Review Board (IRB) of the medical center where the experiment is taking place. The existence and makeup of the IRB, which includes both doctors and laypersons, is mandated by law. The IRB also reviews the consent forms signed by the patients involved.

In addition to the IRB, governmental regulatory agencies like the FDA may also oversee the experiment and have reporting requirements.

These boards and agencies protect the patient from inappropriate experiments. They also help to insure that the experiment is fulfilling its purpose, which is to treat your condition and to generate meaningful information that will lead to treatment decisions for others.

How can you know if you are part of an experiment if you are not told about it? Anytime, for example, that you're asked to be randomized, which means being assigned to a treatment based on chance, you're in an experiment. To put it roughly, if something smells like an experiment, then ask questions until you've gotten enough answers to satisfy your doubts. Ask the surgeon outright: "Is this part of an IRB-approved investigation with informed consent?" If you don't like his answer, get another opinion from a second doctor. If you find out your surgeon is proposing an experimental procedure but not telling you, then it's your choice whether you want to continue with that surgeon.

Outrageous cases do happen, but very rarely. Two plastic surgeons at a very reputable institution were debating about the ways a face-lift should be done. One advocated a more extensive repair technique than the other. They decided to do a test where they did one technique on one side of a patient's face, and the second technique on the other side. They did not tell the patient they were doing this, figuring that if one side was worse than the other, they'd redo it for free.

Stories like this should not make you run away from surgery; instead view them like neon lights, flashing "buyer beware" signs. There are plenty of safeguards built into the system, from your own instincts to the responsibility of doctors and institutions to the laws and regulations of the country.

What often happens is that the media learns of an experimental procedure, then people hear about it and are eager to take advantage of its benefits. Sometimes its acceptance gains speed before enough doctors are experienced in doing it or are confident enough that the risks are understood.

If a procedure is still experimental, the data may be particularly complex and pose a challenge that causes a patient to navigate through sophisticated statistical analysis. She may have to consider questions like: "Is testing on 500 women enough? What is the difference between the methods of conducting, say, a retrospective study versus a randomized prospective study?" For some patients, it may be unfair to try to burden them with the fine points of scientific data; for others, they wouldn't think of going forward without it.

At some point, a physician needs to formulate her own opinion and present it to the patient. When there is an experimental procedure under consideration, as a patient, you want a physician who has the moral conscience only to offer you something that, if not fully validated, she deems to be the best option.

EXPERIENCE AND SKILL

There is a joke that goes around in which the patient asks the doctor, "Have you been successful doing this operation?" When the doctor says, "Yes, I've been successful doing this," that means she's done it once. If she says "I've been successful in case after case," that means she's done it twice.

It may be funny, but it's also a reminder that you need to find out whether your physician truly has a level of skill in a new procedure. If she's done the particular surgery twice, is it okay with you to be the third? Or under your criteria, do you only want a physician who's performed the operation twenty times? Experience in and of itself is not a guarantee of quality, but it is an indication of competency.

Sometimes, a new method has been developed, the benefits are clear, and there is an immediate clamor for it. There can be a rush to perform the procedure and you may find yourself being treated by a surgeon whose training and experience to date consists of watching the operation being done or performing it only under the direction of an expert. Consider whether that is okay with you or if you want to find a surgeon who has advanced her skills through multiple operations. Ask directly, "How many times have you done this surgery yourself? What have the outcomes been?"

If I am considering a new treatment, should I only go to a well-known medical center where a procedure is likely to be done a lot?

Consumers often make decisions on the basis of brand names. And medicine is no different. Well-known medical centers whose names have become brands in the medical community usually developed their reputation for a very good reason. Much, but not all, of the new knowledge in medicine originates in academic hospitals. Often the best community medical centers are also associated to some degree with academic hospitals.

Still, you want to keep in mind that it's the outcome, not the name of the institution that you're after. Look beyond the general reputation of a medical center to its experience with the type of surgery you're considering. Get specific data from the hospital. For example, ask how often the operation is done there. Furthermore, what are the mortality and complication rates associated with that operation at the hospital?

This is the kind of information that a high-quality medical facility should gather. The best institutions, in general, maintain a lot more information than those that are not as good. It is reasonable to expect a hospital to have a quality-control department to collect data about the surgery that takes place within its walls. In addition, that data should be reviewed and analyzed by the management of the hospital—and accessible to a patient who asks for it. It's not that you're just poking around; you're building a case to be confident about going to an institution where you'll be placing your body on the line.

If you are having an experimental or complex treatment, the level of experience of such an institution, confirmed by hard data, may be the deciding factor for you.

Can't I avoid a lot of these difficult questions simply by choosing noninvasive surgery if it's available for my condition?

Make no mistake about it—anything termed noninvasive surgery is still surgery. You are subjecting your body to trauma and you are putting yourself at risk of complications just as you do in surgery that is labeled invasive. That the term "noninvasive surgery" has become so popular should be viewed more as a marketing success than as a way to breeze through surgery.

The reason patients are drawn to so-called noninvasive surgical procedures is that they expect less trauma, less pain, and a quicker recovery than they would have in surgery that requires a larger opening into the body. That may not necessarily be the case for any specific surgery for a particular person. With the exception of a laparoscopic cholecystectomy (removal of the gallbladder), many of these types of surgeries have not been around long enough to know what the long-term outcomes are. All the kinks haven't been worked out yet and there hasn't been enough experience to say with certainty whether, in a given situation, it may be necessary to come back at a later date and have the procedure done again.

It's not that you shouldn't opt for surgery that is called noninvasive if that's the best choice for you. Rather, in the face of hype about what it is, the challenge is to look at such surgery through the same lens that you use to investigate any procedure in which your body is opened up and repaired. In both cases, you have to make a very serious decision and you don't want to cloud what happens during surgery, how recovery unfolds, and whether you get the outcome you want.

MINIMAL-ACCESS SURGERY

Based on what actually happens in the operating room, the term "noninvasive" surgery is better replaced by "minimal-access" surgery.

One increasingly common type of minimal-access surgery uses a scope, or thin, tubular instrument that is inserted into the body through body orifices or very small incisions called ports. For example, an endoscope is used for entering hollow areas like the stomach and an arthroscope goes into joints like the knee. By using these instruments, a surgeon gains access deep into the body. Further, she can see what's going on inside and repair the damage.

Although scopes have been used for decades by urologists and gynecologists, what's different today is that the design of the scopes is far more flexible and the light sources for interior vision have improved dramatically. The surgeon doesn't have to look inside by peering through one eye into a telescope-like device anymore. Instead, scopes carry very small cameras inside the body and send back an image that is projected onto a video screen. Based on those images, the surgeon makes decisions and performs the operation using special instruments that also enter the body through one or more additional ports. She can see what she's doing by watching the video projection.

Many patients have experienced less pain and shorter recovery time from being operated on in this manner. Yet minimal access can also mean minimal visibility. Further, complications can happen, including injury to surrounding tissue. As in any type of surgery, you need to find out what the risks are, including bleeding or infection.

For example, in the earlier days of laparoscopic cholecystectomies, there were many bile-duct injuries and complications from bleeding and infection. As the experience with the technique has grown, the complications have significantly decreased.

Be sure you distinguish the specific minimal-access surgery that you're considering from other types using similar techniques. At what point on the learning curve is the surgery? Has it been done for ten years, with the risks well known, or are you one of the early ones to have the operation, with several unknowns? Can the physician supply you with the data to confirm that this type of surgery will mean less discomfort and fewer complications?

The questions posed by choosing among a set of alternatives are difficult even under the best of circumstances. But when a person is facing an operation for a medical problem, the circumstances can hardly be described as ideal. Emotions are running high, the logistics of managing a life and a treatment course are daunting, and physical pain and weakness are often present.

But you shouldn't be confused, buffeted by one dilemma or another. Instead, put yourself on steady ground, working hand in hand with a competent, caring physician. How do you find a doctor who can listen to you, talk to you, and perform a treatment that will change your life for the better? Read the next chapter.

4

Finding the Right Surgeon

If you're going to have surgery, put this task at the top of your list: find a surgeon who has the skill to understand and repair your problem and who can communicate well.

In the process that stretches from deciding to have an operation to recovering from its effects, your surgeon is the one calling the medical shots. She's at the helm, whether directly during the consultation and surgery, or indirectly through the choices she's made that have an impact on you. For example, a surgeon's hospital affiliation determines where you have your surgery. The staff she's hired become key conduits for your information, support, encouragement, and treatment. The tone that she sets permeates her practice, leading to details like how long you have to wait for appointments to how easily your questions are answered.

COMMUNICATION

A surgeon can, and should, communicate with you in a way that acknowledges you as a person. If a surgeon isn't able to do that, either because of time problems or because she is not as adept at addressing your concerns as you personally need, she should counter that limitation by having other qualified staff in her practice available to sit down and talk with you.

You should feel it is okay to raise topics that are uncomfortable. For example, you might wonder what happens if something unexpected occurs during surgery while you are in a deep sleep. Ask your surgeon what kinds of situations could come up that might require an on-the-spot decision and how she would handle it.

This will help you recognize that during the operation the surgeon has decision-making power over the course of the operation, both the planned and the unexpected. You could compare the experience to flying on an airplane. The pilot does not consult you if there's an emergency decision to be made during the flight. You hand over that authority when you buy your ticket and step on the plane. You are relying on the fact that you've chosen a safe aircraft, a maintenance team who's kept it in shape, controllers who monitor the flight path, and a pilot who knows what to do. You don't even think about or see most of these people.

In surgery, you also are relying on a team, a set of equipment, and a surgeon who is in charge.

Don't go into the operation thinking, "Gee, I wonder if I can talk to somebody about this question I have." Maybe you've held off raising questions because you assumed the surgeon would be too brusque in replying. You've seen television shows where, unlike sensitive-type physicians in other specialties, the surgeons are portrayed as incommunicative technicians. It's one thing to enjoy a good show; but it's another to buy into it as a model in your own life. If you accept without question the caricature of the surgeon as robot, you do a disservice to yourself and your need to know what's happening to you.

By the time you are in the operating room, you've talked to your doctor and her medical staff, read publications, watched videos, and discussed pertinent issues with other patients who've been through it. Now it's time for all of this to bear fruit through an operation. This isn't the end of your questions, since there's still recovery and follow-up to contend with. But, if you did your part at the beginning, you shouldn't have the question, "Why did I have this operation?"

Throughout the preceding chapters, I have referred to the key role of the physician at various points in the decision-making process. In this chapter, I pull together those threads to create the patchwork of information and inspiration that allows you to put yourself, confidently, in the hands of your surgeon.

YOUR ROLE

Don't expect to sit with your arms folded, watching someone else restore you to health. You have an active role to play in the primary medical relationship you have with your surgeon.

Be candid. Tell the doctor what it is you really want, what you fear, what concerns you. Focus on the issues critical to information gathering and decision making. If you need open-heart surgery, don't spend an hour talking about your childhood hay fever.

Honor your commitments and stick with the agenda. Be straight-forward and tell your doctor when you're having problems following through on any pre-op instructions. If you have a heart condition and your surgeon has recommended surgery *and* a restricted diet, it doesn't help either of you if you hide the fact that you haven't been staying on the eating plan.

Identify a reasonable number of family members, significant others, or friends with whom the doctor should communicate. Recognize how difficult it is for the doctor if twenty people are calling independently each day after surgery for an update.

PERCEPTIONS

There is a wide range of medical problems capable of being treated by surgery. The lens through which you view your choice of surgeon depends in part on where your condition falls on that spectrum.

If you're doing something relatively routine, like having your appendix out, it isn't likely you'll have a sustained relationship with your surgeon. You will probably see her only once more in a post-surgical visit.

On the other hand, if you're having breast cancer surgery, your emotional well-being is critical. You're looking for someone who is sensitive to the impact the disease has on you and who will also be the captain of a complicated medical ship. You're not just facing an operation, but also a long post-operative program that potentially involves chemotherapy and radiation. It is reasonable to expect to have a surgeon who is not just going to perform the surgery and be done with you, but one who will have a continuing role in your treatment.

There are many ways to find a surgeon and evaluate her. But even hard data gets filtered through your perceptions. It helps to explore what ideas you have about what a surgeon is and does. You can evaluate whether those thoughts make sense when you see yourself not just as a patient, but also as an informed consumer about to hire a skilled professional to perform a serious job.

Trust

In the operation itself, the surgeon is following through on your mutual agreement: you lie still and she'll inflict real trauma on your body, albeit through accepted medical protocol. When you enter into that kind of contract, you better be very sure it's for a good reason and with a person who knows just what to do.

That level of trust you feel is bolstered by external facts about another person like recommendations, certifications, and experience. Your instinct plays a big role here; you need to tap into it and trust it. If you have a negative feeling about a doctor after you consult with her or if something doesn't seem quite right to you about the diagnosis and proposed treatment, don't just dismiss your reaction. Use it as an incentive to investigate further.

No one says this is easy. Sometimes you learn from hindsight what instincts you should have heeded. A woman who had a painful abscess in a gland in the labia had to find a gynecologist to treat the condition. The patient's usual gynecologist, a solo practitioner whose office was in her old hometown, was away for two weeks. Since the patient had recently moved to a new town, she called the only local doctor she knew, her husband's internist. He gave her the name of the biggest gynecological practice in town.

The lack of good feeling about the doctor started when the patient first met the gynecologist. From the start she felt the doctor was competent, especially since she was part of the community's largest practice. But she didn't like the doctor's rushed manner, her brusque way of drawing a picture of the problem on the paper that covers the examining table, or her long discussion about payment arrangements when she didn't have time to spend on a slower discussion of medical matters. Nevertheless, the patient followed her recommendations.

The doctor tried to lance the abscess in the office. It was extremely painful and didn't work. Then she suggested surgery after a few days of antibiotic treatment. The surgery required thirty stitches and the patient was in great pain for several days afterward. She had to call the doctor because she didn't have enough painkillers. She wasn't told either by the doctor or her staff that extreme pain could last as long as six days and that her range of motion could be restricted for that time.

About three weeks after the surgery, the abscess returned. The patient called the gynecologist who said another surgery might be necessary and to come in for an appointment. At that point, the patient decided she'd had enough, called her original gynecologist who was now back in his office, and went the fifty miles for the appointment. It was worth it to her. He spent an adequate amount of time with her, confirmed that the condition was extremely painful, explained why lancing was an unnecessary and painful intervention, and prescribed a regimen of hot baths and antibiotics. The abscess went away and a second surgery wasn't necessary.

What could this patient have done differently to prevent some of the hassles she went through? By dismissing the condition as relatively minor in the scheme of things—it was an abscess and not a tumor—she didn't take many precautions in choosing a doctor. Even though she was new in town, she realized she could have made some effort to find out the doctor's reputation among patients. That way she might have found out before, rather than after, that this was a doctor who was not particularly sensitive to a patient's pain threshold.

Although the lancing episode was almost unbearable, she didn't heed that warning to question whether the doctor would be forthcoming about pain after surgery. Also, the patient didn't do any independent research, like going on the Internet, to find out more about the condition (which she had never heard of before). If she had taken these steps, she thinks she would have been on more solid ground to question the doctor's recommendations. She didn't let her annoyance at the doctor's manner provoke her to evaluate whether this was the right doctor for her.

When you are having any surgery, especially one that's relatively minor, you may be tempted to just accept a recommendation, be lax about asking questions, and ignore your instincts. Even minor surgery, however, can be a major matter for your body.

The patient said she still believes the gynecologist was technically competent, but she wouldn't go back to her because she doesn't trust her level of empathy or interest in providing a patient with a thorough, unhurried explanation—or a complete picture of what to expect in the aftermath of surgery. A recommendation from another doctor, a busy practice, or a list of credentials cannot tell you whether a doctor has the outlook and sensitivity you need to make your surgical experience as bearable as possible. Those are things you glean from your personal encounter with a physician and you would do well to heed them. Do you prefer a doctor with a crisp edge or a soft manner? You should feel comfortable with the way the doctor talks to you and the way the doctor examines you. Your response to those gestures is an indicator of whether this is the right doctor for you.

Don't drive yourself crazy analyzing a doctor's behavior, but don't shortchange yourself either. If your instincts are knocking loudly, at least open the door to them and see what they have to say.

WHAT TO LOOK FOR IN A SURGEON

- *Skill in treating the disease you have.* Find out how many operations the surgeon has performed personally in the *specific* type of surgery you're facing. It's a fair question and the information should be readily available.

- *Responsiveness to your needs.* You say you are nervous about anesthesia. Does your surgeon ignore the comment or does she (or a designated staff member) take the time to discuss anesthesia in detail with you? Does she give you printed information, outline what choices you have, and tell you what to expect in your pre-operative anesthesia evaluation?

- *Ability to inspire confidence.* Does the accumulated information and experience that you've gathered about a surgeon lead you to trust that surgeon?

Star Quality

Perceived wisdom is that if you hire a star, a person who has name recognition, you'll have success. Reputations of star surgeons are, in fact, usually well deserved. Their recognition tends to come either from having a very large, broad-based practice in a community or from being known as a leader in their field because of innovation or technical prowess.

There is at least some hard evidence to back up the reasoning behind hiring a "brand-name" surgeon. Typically, well-known surgeons get more referrals, see more patients, and as a result, do more surgeries. In one reliable source of data, a study of the mortality rates in coronary bypass surgery listed by individual surgeons in New York state, the results show that the mortality rates of patients are lower for surgeons whose volume of surgery is higher.

Patients, of course, do not land in a doctor's office because of some kind of anonymous steering mechanism. They end up seeing a surgeon because they've been referred by a word-of-mouth system of recommendation, which draws heavily on a surgeon's reputation in a given field.

The concern is sometimes raised that a star surgeon means a too-busy surgeon who is likely to brush off questions. Don't buy into that. The star surgeon can take the time to answer questions to put a patient at ease and will also have a support staff available to answer questions.

On the other hand, have you ever watched a sports team put all its money into hiring a super athlete, only to lose the championship because the rest of the team doesn't match up? One thing to be aware of when you are seeking out the best names in the field is whether you are also getting the qualities of a topnotch institution: considerate treatment and a compassionate staff, from your first pre-op visit to your last post-surgical visit.

Sometimes a medical facility will put all its efforts into hiring a marquee name only to neglect the other aspects of the surgical experience. A top surgeon was recently offered a leadership position at an institution that not only had a number of brand-name physicians on its staff, but also an internationally renowned pioneer in surgery. When the visiting surgeon was considering the position, he was appalled to find that the systems supporting those names were primitive by the standards of the 1990s. The surgeon decided not to take the job.

You may well want to go to the biggest name in the field in your location; or you may even be willing to travel some distance. This may be especially important if you are having a risky, complicated, or unusual procedure. If you're having fairly routine surgery, you should look for a surgeon who may not be in the record books, but has done many of the same type of surgery you are going to have and is known among her peers and her patients as being competent and caring.

Surgical Style

Try not to make a decision based only on a surgeon's style. Pinning facile phrases on a surgeon, such as conservative, aggressive, or "knife-happy," is not a helpful approach.

Descriptive labels like conservative or aggressive can mean different things to different people. Be very clear about what's being discussed when these words are bandied about. Take the example of performing hip surgery on a very old person. It's a big operation with significant risk, yet there is a plausible argument that surgical treatment of a hip fracture in an elderly patient is conservative therapy. The alternative, confining an elderly person to bed, can be considered the more aggressive approach. In this case you've made an even more radical decision than surgery. You've given up on a person's ability ever to walk again.

Words like aggressive or conservative cloud the real issues you need to consider. Instead of using meaningless labels, state what you are looking for in a direct way: "I want a surgeon who follows the most effective course for treating the disease with the lowest risk of complications." Or say, "I want a surgeon who can cure this thing, even if she has to apply a cutting-edge technique that still has a lot of questions surrounding it." What you don't want is to discover, in retrospect, that you've gone through an operation you wish you hadn't had done because of a misunderstanding or stereotyping.

HOW TO FIND A SURGEON

One of the most common ways to find a surgeon is to get a recommendation from a physician you know, like your primary-care doctor. You can put the question to her in a direct, personal way: "If you were having this type of abdominal surgery, which surgeon would be your first choice to do the operation?" Doctors expect questions like this, and as a matter of course, refer patients to surgeons.

What if you are concerned that your doctor is not being objective, that she is referring you to someone not necessarily because she's the best surgeon but because she's a friend? You don't have to squelch the little cynical voices inside you. Instead, make them even louder voices. Ask another doctor, or two or three, who they would recommend as a surgeon. If you're getting consistent answers that point to the initial recommendation, then you can feel comfortable with it. If not, you'll probably want to look further.

How do doctors know who's good? As professionals they are part of a network. Doctors certainly do talk among themselves and share information. They also have one of the best resources available to evaluate surgeons—feedback from patients they already referred. Through direct, first-hand accounts, doctors find out on a very basic level how a surgeon works, whether a patient was satisfied or not, and what the surgical outcome was. A caring physician is going to use that information in determining whether to refer a surgeon to the next patient who needs an operation.

If a doctor doesn't know someone in a certain specialty or location, she generally knows a colleague to call who does. Furthermore, doctors are adept at using resources to find references within their profession.

You can seek recommendations from nonphysicians whom you believe to be knowledgeable. This is a judgment call on your part. Your aunt who works in administration at the local hospital probably would be a good resource. Who among your circle of family and friends might be a good source of a referral for you?

When you get a recommendation, be sure to ask why as well as who. A woman got a recommendation for a doctor from someone she knew. When she went to the appointment, she hated the doctor. Only later she found out that her acquaintance was agoraphobic (unusually fearful of going outdoors) and the reason she liked the doctor was because her office was around the corner.

There are innumerable resources available to you from which you can obtain the name of a surgeon, including: organizations of medical professionals, like the American College of Surgeons, or rosters maintained by high-quality hospitals. (See the Resources section at the end of this book.) Such listings lack the nuance of a personal recommendation. However, they do point you in the direction of a surgeon whom the medical community deems competent, either through employment at a respected institution or by inclusion in a medical directory that carefully screens its data.

Experience

How much is enough for you? Do you want someone who has performed a hundred surgeries of a certain type? Or is someone who has more recently finished medical training a better candidate in your mind? Some people prefer a surgeon who has years under her belt; others feel that a newly trained surgeon is more likely to be current with the latest techniques.

How much experience makes for a good surgeon may be a question mark; data on it, as expressed by number of years in practices and surgeries performed, is available to any patient who requests it.

When a ninety-one-year-old woman fell off her bed, she landed in the hospital with a broken hip. She was trying to decide between not having surgery, which likely meant not being able to walk again, and having an operation that would enable her to walk but would subject her to the risks of complications that are greater for a woman her age. Her nephew asked the surgeon, "How many successful hip operations have you done on people my aunt's age?" Both the patient and her family were reassured to find out not only had the surgeon done almost a thousand hip surgeries, but more than fifty of them had been on patients older than ninety. This kind of information helped make it easier to decide to have the surgery.

When you're looking at numbers, it's important that the surgeon doesn't just describe statistics about the surgery from textbooks and articles or tell you about how many of these operations *another* surgeon has done. There can be a disparity between the statistics from the surgeon or hospital you're using and those from an ideal setting.

It doesn't mean a surgeon is hiding something if she doesn't maintain a lot of statistical information. But a surgeon should be able to describe her history and identify the types and frequency of complications that she's encountered.

In choosing a surgeon, sometimes you can't go by a title alone. For example, if you are going to have thyroid surgery, you may be referred to a general surgeon, an ear, nose, and throat surgeon, a head and neck surgeon, or a plastic surgeon. One of the simplest questions to ask if the doctor's specialty confuses you is: "How many of these procedures have you done?"

Numbers aren't the only factor that count. Consider also that the great new surgeons of the future have to begin at some point. It may happen that your illness is not improving under known therapies done by reputable surgeons in the field. You may hear of a new surgeon who takes a different approach. Do you feel confident enough in the surgeon's skills and the method she advocates to put yourself in her hands?

That was the question that faced a man several years ago who had recurrent abscesses on his lower back. He went through multiple operations to get rid of them, yet the abscesses returned. When he was planning to have yet another operation by one of the major surgeons in New York, his wife suggested he see a young surgeon who posed a completely different solution to the problem. The man had never heard of this physician before, but the surgeon explained the procedure, and what it could do for him, thoughtfully and rationally. Since the other operations had not been successful, he decided to go for it. The new kid on the block solved the problem—and went on to become one of the preeminent surgeons in his field.

So, faced with the choice of staying in the comfort zone where a longtime surgeon has done the same procedure in the same way for years or stepping outside of it to go with a new surgeon and a new technique, how do you decide? Questions to consider include:

Does the new surgeon's approach make sense to you?
How does it match up with the information you've reviewed from other sources?

Has she built up a reputation so far?
Is she associated with a high-quality medical center?
Do you have confidence based on the way the surgeon has communicated the new approach?

DATA

There is clearly something powerful about a personal recommendation. When a person says to you, "I think Dr. X is the best heart surgeon in the city," she is giving you the benefit of her individual experience and an opportunity to ask more questions.

But that type of recommendation isn't always available to you. You may want to back up someone else's opinion with additional facts. In the information age that we live in, there is no need to be ignorant about your doctor's education and history. It can be hard to pin down whether a person shows a caring nature, but it is not hard to find out whether she has credentials. Where did she go to medical school, is she board-certified, has she been involved in a malpractice suit? Has she done research that's been published or been honored by awards or fellowships?

If you feel the choice of who performs your surgery calls for the kind of investigation that, say, you would put into buying a computer, then be assured the information is out there in one form or another. A résumé written by the doctor, a certification issued by a distinguished medical board, a mention in an annual review of "best doctors" by a reputable publication, a record of the number of surgeries performed by the doctor as maintained by the medical center where she practices is available, waiting for you to retrieve it.

Education

The need to know a doctor's credentials is important, but asking for that information is often a luxury there isn't enough time for in office visits. That's one good reason for doctors to hang their diplomas on the wall for you to view. You can also call the surgeon's office and ask that a biography or résumé be sent to you.

You can go to the library and ask the reference librarian to show you the appropriate medical reference books. In books like the *Directory of Physicians in the U.S.,* published by the American Medical Association, you can find doctors listed alphabetically and by geographic location. The book supplies basic information and is a comprehensive way to start your research.

Certification

Medical boards are organizations in the U.S. that set standards for training and continued education in medicine. Board certification assures patients that a physician has successfully passed rigorous review. There are about twenty-four medical boards and they include specialties in general surgery and in specific fields like colon and rectal surgery.

At a minimum, you want to be operated on by a board-certified surgeon. That information should be easily attainable from your doctor. You can also look up which doctors are certified and in which specialties in *The Official ABMS Directory of Board-Certified Medical Specialists.* ABMS stands for the American Board of Medical Specialists. The directory is available in book form, on CD-ROM, and on-line. Insurance-company directories also indicate whether a physician is certified in a particular field.

Other Published Data

Some states publish data in different formats that you may, or may not, find useful in your research. New York State, for example, has put out a report for several years called "Coronary Artery Bypass Surgery." It lists, by medical center and by surgeon's name, the number of patients who died during this type of surgery or shortly after. It gives you one endpoint—survival rate—and compares it to the norm.

Other states publish reports on surgeons' credentials and whether any malpractice suits have been filed. You can find out what information your state collects and publishes by calling your state's board of medicine or health department.

Medical societies or organizations that deal with a specific disease are also a good resource. For instance, if you have inflammatory bowel disease, your doctor's office will provide you with the phone number of an association that collects information on that disease and you can find out from them which hospitals and physicians are well known in the field.

The popular press also publishes a great deal of medical information, including lists of the "best" physicians in a given geographic area based on their own research. These lists can serve not only as a guide to identify surgeons, but also to highlight the types of issues and questions independent journalists use to evaluate doctors.

Each publication has its own method of finding the doctors they are highlighting. For example, researchers may call a number of doctors and ask them to review a list of physicians who are not part of their own institution and answer the following question for each one: "Would you want a family member of yours taken care of by this doctor?"

If the publication is reputable, you can expect it to be a reasonable resource for finding a doctor. But don't give up on your doctor if she isn't on the list. The names of lots of very good physicians never turn up on such published lists.

EVALUATING A SURGEON

- *Speak directly with the surgeon.* This is your opportunity for first-hand research. After you've had time to mull over the consultation, do you come away with a good feeling about this surgeon?

- *Examine her credentials.* Where did the surgeon go to medical school and where did she do her residency? Is she certified by a medical board in the specialty that treats your problem?

- *Find out the surgeon's reputation in the medical community.* Your referring doctor is an initial source for this information. You can check further by calling another doctor you know to see if she concurs.

- *Consider the hospital where the surgeon practices.* Is it one that is well respected in your community?

- *Ask the opinion of nurses.* They work with many doctors and often know who is respected and who is not.

- *Ask at the surgeon's office if the surgeon has been recognized in print or in "best doctor" lists published in magazines and books.* Surely not a prerequisite for choosing a doctor, yet it is helpful to know how the surgeon has been regarded by the media.

CONSULTATION WITH A SURGEON

Asking questions is a big part of the process of understanding your surgery, who is going to do it, and how. After all, this is unfamiliar territory to you. When you enter a surgeon's office for a consultation, expect to hear an understandable, coherent explanation of the following:

- Your medical problem.

- What results you can reasonably expect from an operation.

- The risks of this surgery.

- What you will experience during the operation.

- What will happen during recovery.

In addition, try to find out what kinds of questions other people ask surgeons. Think about what you want to know. Don't waste time with questions you don't care about or already know the answers to. And don't shortchange yourself because you feel timid about talking about what's on your mind. Ask about the basics, then ask the unusual. If it is a concern, then raise the question. Don't be repressed, but be reasonable. You need to recognize that you are not the only patient the doctor will see that day.

Who will do the actual surgery?

You may have heard stories about cases where the surgeon did not actually do the surgery; instead, it was performed by residents. If you have any doubts on this score or have a horror story from a friend that troubles you, don't get as far as the operating room still wondering who is going to remove your gallbladder. Raise the question directly with your surgeon. Will she be performing the entire operation? If she is assisted by residents and colleagues, what parts of the surgery will they do?

No responsible surgeon will turn her work, and the ultimate accountability for that work, over to someone else. But that doesn't mean that others will not be participating in the operation.

During the operation, your surgeon ought to be the captain of the ship. If you believe that surgeon should not be assisted by residents or colleagues and should do all the surgical procedures herself, then you are entitled to say that. By raising the question, you might be opening the door to a discussion that could help you avoid misunderstandings about what happens in an operation.

Your surgeon might tell you it is her belief that the surgeon in charge should not do everything and that good surgeons have good systems in place to help them. She may tell you that the professionals who assist her are extensions of herself, that they are residents and colleagues who have trained together and who share high-performance standards and expectations. By having help, the chief surgeon is free to do the most important parts of the surgery.

If you object to this, it is your choice not to use the surgeon. If you have strong feelings about this topic, or any other with regard to your surgery, ask well in advance, when there is still time to change surgeons if you are not happy with the answers. Be open to changing any misconceptions you may have, and to changing the surgeon if you simply do not agree with a doctor's method of operating. If it is very important to you not to have a resident as part of your surgical team, then you probably shouldn't select a teaching hospital. But don't wait until you're about to have anesthesia to ask the question.

Who is on the surgeon's staff?

Of course your goal is to find a competent, caring surgeon to perform surgery so that you achieve the outcome you want. But no surgeon functions all alone. She has an experienced staff to rely on in her office, during testing, and throughout surgery and recovery.

It is highly likely that many of your questions will not be answered by the surgeon herself, but by medical professionals—the nurse, nurse practitioner, or physician's assistant—who are key members of a surgeon's team.

You have the right to expect that the surgeon's staff will provide the following:

- Courteous treatment.

- Additional information for understanding your condition (e.g., brochures and referrals to support services) and assistance in arranging treatment (directions on how to follow through on setting up appointments, etc.).

If you haven't been to a hospital in a while, you may not have met physician's assistants (PAs) and nurse practitioners before. (See pages 14 and 15 for definitions and education requirements.) They are increasingly becoming significant resources for information and treatment. Though they differ in their training and in what they are licensed to do, both are educated medical professionals who supplement the work of the doctor to a highly skilled extent.

Make it a point to meet the physician's assistants and nurse practitioners who will participate in treating you. This may happen in the doctor's office at the time of your consultation or in the hospital after you've been admitted.

Either one may have extensive discussions with you, perform a range of procedures on you, and prescribe medicine, which they are authorized to do. Nurse practitioners have more freedom to prescribe and may work on their own; PAs work under a doctor's supervision. Nurse practitioners are more likely to be found in internal medicine; PAs are often involved in surgery. For example, if you are having a coronary bypass procedure, a PA with a specialty in surgery may also be in the operating room. She may be removing veins from your legs to be used for the bypass at the same time the surgeon is opening up the chest to get to the heart.

Before the surgery, you should also expect to meet the anesthesiologist, or if the logistics don't work out, a colleague or representative for the anesthesiologist. Your first encounter with the anesthesia department will likely be at the time of your presurgical testing appointment. You will also meet the anesthesiologist again just before your operation.

And of course, throughout your surgical experience, you will have contact with nurses, from the first moments of arriving for a consultation through your departure from the hospital. There are nurses who work in your surgeon's office, and they are a significant resource. They answer your questions, perform procedures like drawing blood, schedule the dates for the operation and pre-surgical testing, and help route you through the entire process.

You will also have substantial contact with other nurses who are employed by the hospital, including nurses on the hospital floor and in the operating room. Nurses are an essential part, along with the surgeon and anesthesiologist, of an operating team. Operating-room nurses are employees of the hospital, not of the surgeon. However, surgeons standardly request the team of nurses with whom they've successfully worked and whom they trust. Part of hiring a surgeon is the realization that you are also signing on for the systems and the staff who work along with that surgeon.

Will the surgeon be providing the post-operative care or is it delegated to somebody else?

Many patients have an image of what the surgeon's continuing role will be after surgery only to be disappointed by a much different reality. Don't expect to have the senior surgeon come in every day to dress your wound or to answer all the questions from you and your family. It's not that the surgeon isn't caring for you; rather, in the normal course of her practice those tasks are handled by another medical professional.

For instance, some heart surgeons may say, "I'll be doing the operation and I'll let you know how things go. But on a day-to-day basis, the person you'll speak with is a cardiologist." Or a surgeon may say a major resource for information and care in her practice after surgery is her physician's assistant. Rather than be disappointed or confused, find out just what to expect.

For routine matters, each surgeon has her own method of delegating responsibilities to other professionals such as medical-specialty colleagues, physician's assistants, or nurses. If you have an unusual problem after surgery, however, you should expect to receive a direct response from the surgeon.

Other staff will be handling your IVs and dressing your wound. The specific skills of a surgeon are not put to best use on those tasks.

Nor should you expect a surgeon to be available any time of the day or night to answer questions that can be very competently handled by other staff.

But that doesn't mean your surgeon should just disappear from view once the operation is over. There should be ongoing contact, preferably on a daily basis. No matter which member of the hospital staff or post-surgical team treats you, the ultimate accountability is the surgeon's.

Where does the surgeon perform the surgery?

Find out if the surgeon practices in an academic center or a community hospital, and learn what the differences are. In some cases, a surgeon may practice at both and you have a choice of where to have your surgery.

An *academic center* usually has the advantage of being able to apply new therapies and advanced treatment techniques and is able to provide a greater depth of service. By definition, an academic hospital has teaching responsibilities that create a system in which the surgeon's work is being scrutinized on a daily basis by medical professionals in training. It also means there will be students and residents who are learning from you as the subject.

Some people don't mind this at all. Others do. Ask your surgeon to describe specifically what it means in your case to be operated on in a teaching hospital. Although it is almost impossible to extricate yourself entirely from the teaching aspect in an academic center, speak to the surgeon if any of this upsets you.

At a *community hospital* you are likely to have the benefit of being in a more intimate setting closer to home. It is reasonable to expect that the quality of routine surgery at a community hospital is high, but that quality does vary from institution to institution. Discuss any question about the reputation of the hospital where the surgery will be performed with the surgeon.

The major focus of the two types of hospitals is different. A teaching hospital focuses on teaching and research; a community hospital on taking care of patients. But there's no reason that a good center can't combine characteristics of both. A good academic institution should also provide a high level of patient care. And a good community hospital should have state-of-the-art techniques and a level of scrutiny that ensures quality medical treatment.

What about the price of the surgery? Is there any flexibility there?

It depends. To the extent you're covered by insurance, such as Medicare or through an HMO, the price has already been set. If you have regular health insurance, then your insurance company will typically pay the usual and customary charges of the surgeon.

If you're paying for anything out-of-pocket, then it is reasonable to consider that you can discuss those costs with your doctor. If you feel uncomfortable about that, recall when you last bought a car. Did you negotiate? Discussing those fees need not be an embarrassment. Rather it's an opportunity to find out where you will end up on the spectrum that goes from having the charges waived to paying the amount in full.

You can also discuss how you pay. Some surgeons' offices will arrange for monthly billing rather than requiring you to pay all at once.

Remember, the cost of the surgeon is not the only cost of surgery. You will have a separate bill from the hospital and you may also have other bills from services that are not part of the hospital charges, such as anesthesiologists, private-duty nursing, laboratory charges, and pathology charges.

Ultimately, the choice of a surgeon is an exercise in finding the right person to operate, who will pull together all the other pieces of the picture—the staff, the directives, the method, and location of the operation—in a way that is best for you.

Part Two, which follows, details the logistics of preparing for your operation, being admitted to the hospital, undergoing your surgery, and remaining for the post-operative hospital stay.

Part Two

BEFORE, DURING, AND AFTER: OPTIMIZING YOUR HOSPITAL STAY

5

Getting Yourself Ready for Surgery

You've made the big decisions about surgery—why you're having it and who's going to do it. You've gone past the point of indecision and second-guessing. Now you can tackle the next steps to help make those medical decisions work for you. These include strengthening yourself physically and mentally, delegating home and work responsibilities, and preparing for unlikely worst-case scenarios.

TAKING CARE OF YOURSELF
Diet, Exercise, and Lifestyle

Doctors have a reputation for being notoriously inattentive to what a patient eats. But that's no reason to assume your own doctor isn't aware, concerned, and informed about nutrition and nutritional supplements like vitamins and minerals.

Why bother with food now? Because you need all the strength your body can muster to absorb the trauma of surgery, fight off infection, and heal well. Studies have shown that a substantial percentage of surgical patients are malnourished.

Before surgery, anxiety and discomfort may turn you off food. During the operation and in the hours, sometimes days, surrounding it, your body is intentionally starved. As you recover, it can be hard physically and emotionally to eat. The effects of anesthesia lessen your appetite, pain medication depresses it, your tubes, dressings, and stitches are irritating, and you can't move your bowels normally. A few weeks ago, your favorite meal of garlicky tomato sauce over pasta, fresh salad, and bread out of the oven might have been a real pleasure. Right now, the thought of it, let alone its taste and smell, is nauseating.

Sure, you'll get sustenance if you need it through your veins or by means of a tube in your intestinal tract. But you can't just rely on stopgap measures to replace the nutrients that are being depleted during the course of having and recovering from surgery.

Where do you get solid information on how to connect your nutritional needs to your healing process? Hardly a day goes by without new data being published in the popular press about food and supplements. However, the information is sometimes contradictory and confusing. Be aware that there are safety issues with nutritional supplements and vitamins. Considering the use of any product as a therapy is not much different from analyzing the benefits versus the risks of an operation or a prescription drug.

Your doctor already has basic indicators like weight, height, and blood tests that can identify your nutritional status. Start your questions here, but if your doctor is not skilled in nutrition, ask him to refer you to a registered dietitian or nutritionist. A registered dietitian has satisfied credentialing tests, including fulfilling continuing education requirements; a nutritionist does not have to fulfill the same stringent requirements.

Nutrition professionals can answer questions such as when you should add supplements like zinc and vitamin C and whether you'd benefit more from a protein-rich diet or one high in carbohydrates in the days before surgery. They would look at these topics in the context of your own nutritional makeup and the type of surgery you're having.

Do you really need to consult a professional about diet at this time? No. Basic common sense can lead you to eat healthy foods and take a multivitamin to support your body in healing and fighting off infection. To stay in shape before surgery, stay balanced. If anxiety affects your eating patterns, try to avoid the extremes of eating too much or too little. Sometimes smaller, more frequent meals are a more comfortable way to eat.

If you are having gastrointestinal surgery, normal eating patterns will be a long way off. If your foot is going to be operated on, your return to three-course meals will be a lot quicker. It's important to recognize no matter what surgery you're having, what you eat and drink is one weapon in an arsenal of many to help you fight your way back to health.

You may have dietary issues that go beyond strengthening yourself for surgery, and relate to some of your core medical problems. A low-fat diet might be mandatory if you are going to make a long-term recovery from coronary artery disease. If you've been operated on for colon cancer, consider what you eat when you work on preventing recurrence. If cholesterol is a problem for you, some hospitals have preventive medicine divisions that concentrate on helping you eat a low-fat, low-cholesterol diet. If necessary, a physician can prescribe cholesterol-lowering medication.

Eating happens to be something people really enjoy and if they have to adopt a very stringent diet, they're miserable. But if someone's had three heart attacks and a cholesterol level of 400, I think he had better change his eating habits no matter how little fun it is. On the other hand, if a man is eighty-two and has had an active lifestyle, his first episode of angina doesn't mean he's got to go vegetarian.

Exercise is also a way to strengthen your body. If you've been exercising all along, keep it up if your doctor agrees. Tell him what you typically do and ask if those motions could have a negative impact on the type of operation you're going to have. Running a marathon is not a good idea at this time, but walking or bike riding might be. In some cases, like before a coronary bypass operation, you may need to restrict your activity so you don't precipitate symptoms or a heart attack. After surgery, review your exercise program with your doctor and decide when, and at what level, you can resume it.

Is this a time to try new things? For some people, a medical crisis leads them to dig in and stay put. For others, it's one of those turning points in life when they seek change. Even if you've never tried it before, eating more vegetables, doing a daily vitamin regimen, and taking up an exercise like yoga or tai chi might appeal to you now.

The Night Before Surgery

Always make sure to follow the particular instructions your doctor gives you. The general rule is you do not eat or drink anything after midnight on the night before surgery because you are going to have anesthesia the next day. One of the potentially fatal risks of anesthesia is the possibility that you could vomit the contents of your stomach and suck them into your trachea and lungs. It is for very good reason that elective surgery done under general anesthesia is performed only on a patient with an empty stomach.

In some cases, your doctor may allow you to have clear liquids like water or apple juice on the day of surgery. You may also be able to have some water if you are taking medication by mouth. Little sips of water before surgery are generally not considered a risk in terms of anesthesia, but don't assume that is true in your case.

Restricted Diet Due to Medical Problems

There are many different reasons why your doctor may put you on a regimen of dietary restrictions, either immediately before surgery or in a time period leading up to surgery. These include:

- *Medical conditions such as obesity or diabetes:* If you are seriously overweight, your doctor may direct you to lose a number of pounds before surgery. If a very heavy person needs a coronary bypass operation, there is an increased risk of complications from removing the veins needed for the bypass from that patient's legs if they are very large and fluid-filled. Surgery may even be postponed until the weight comes down to a safer level.

  Some large hospitals have centers devoted to the care and management of patients with diabetes, where specially trained professionals teach patients about topics like how to manage diabetes when they are having surgery.

- *Requirements of the surgery itself:* Certain types of surgery may have instructions about what you eat or drink that are specifically connected to the nature of the operation. For example, if you are having intestinal surgery you may be required to go through a pre-surgical intestinal cleansing routine.

Beneficial Health Changes

As you focus on the part of the body being operated on, do not neglect the rest of your health. If you have any poor habits, working on them beforehand may help ease your recovery from surgery. If you are still smoking, ideally you should stop at least a month before a scheduled operation. Smoking makes a big difference in your postoperative state. You are likely to have more phlegm, coughing, and more pain when you do cough. The complication of pneumonia is much more frequent in smokers.

Just the recognition—and the fear—that you are increasing the likelihood of major complications is a significant inducement to go cold turkey, at least for the brief period in the weeks before surgery. If you need help to stop smoking, talk to your surgeon about aids like nicotine patches, medication, or hypnosis.

Medications, Vitamins, and Other Supplements

Your medical professional is the only guide to what medicines you should take and when to take them. So be sure your doctor knows all the prescription drugs you are taking. When you first saw your surgeon, you filled out a questionnaire listing those drugs. If you're not sure you've included everything, or if anything has changed, ask to go over the list. Don't judge on your own whether something is insignificant or not.

The same goes for nonprescription drugs. Just because you bought a drug over-the-counter doesn't mean it isn't powerful or its effect can't be altered when it's taken in combination with other medicines. Describe all nonprescription drugs that you're taking to your doctor. Certain ones, like aspirin or ibuprofen, generally have to be stopped before surgery. These drugs are blood thinners that may lead to excessive bleeding during surgery.

Tell your doctor *anything* you are taking as medicine, and that includes vitamins, herbs, or other substances that you don't think of as medicine. For example, some vitamins can counteract blood-thinning medications. Your doctor needs to know what you are taking so he can advise you whether to continue or to stop.

Responsibilities

Maybe you've never been incapacitated. People have always depended on you to do everything. If you don't know where to start to get help, begin by asking at your doctor's office. Their primary function is not to find care for your family while you're in the hospital, but to point you toward resources you may need. Your doctor's office works with the hospital's social-work department, which has lists of recommended child-care agencies, home health aids, and other services you may need while hospitalized. When you leave the hospital, social workers will work out a plan with you for your care. This will be discussed in detail in Chapter 6.

Depending on your illness and its treatment, you may only need to delegate a few days' worth of work at the office—or you may need to take a leave of absence. Handling the affairs of your job is your own business, but if you need help convincing the boss that you really will be out of commission, let the medical staff know what kind of obstacles you're encountering. Your doctor or a social worker can provide a letter to your boss and to your insurance company verifying your surgery and hospital stay, if you are requesting disability insurance.

Personal issues are often a very important part of a patient's decision to have an operation, or more commonly, when to have it. Doctors often hear patients say that having an operation would pose an undue burden on their family. If the issue is having a face-lift at the same time your young child is anxious about starting a new school or your elderly mother is ill and needs your supervision, then it may not make sense to do it now. On the other hand, if you're having surgery to remove a cancerous section of your colon, don't put it off because you think someone else needs you more. This is a time to put yourself first.

All the exercise and good food in the world won't keep your

strength up if you sap your energy with worries. Don't pack a stack of bills that need to be paid in your suitcase for the hospital. Don't start tracking down baby-sitters for your kids once your hospital phone is installed. And don't plan to conclude that big deal at work from your hospital bed.

Don't bring your outside troubles with you, but do consider how you'll deal with them when you leave. The time to start your discharge planning is before you get to the hospital. This step is relevant for all types of surgery, but it is particularly important to those who have a complicated operation or a complicated social situation. If you have any concerns, it is perfectly appropriate to ask to see the social worker beforehand. Either your surgeon can refer you, or you can call on your own initiative.

Make as many arrangements as you can so that whoever, and whatever, has a claim on your time can be put off until you're well enough to take up your tasks again. If ever there was a reason to call on your support network of family and friends, this is it.

A woman who broke both legs in a car accident had surgery to repair them, was in the hospital for two weeks, and then returned home to recuperate for a few months. Three years later, she elected to have a second operation to remove the pins and plates because they had become so painful. She decided to have the surgery at Christmas when her business was quiet. It's a lesson she learned from the previous time when she couldn't choose to make her surgery fit her schedule. This woman owns her own consulting firm and some clients went elsewhere permanently when she couldn't handle their matters during her surgery and recuperation. Try to tell your business associates in advance that you will not be available. Most people are sympathetic, but you can't prevent some losses when you're not at the helm.

You may be pleasantly surprised by how many people *will* be willing to help you, as this patient discovered. She belongs to several community groups, and on their own initiative, members from those organizations—people she didn't know personally—had prepared food and delivered it. If you belong to a group, whether it's a church, school, or a civic or social organization, let them know you're going to be out of commission for a while. They may help you with meals or drive your kids to lessons after school. If this makes you uncomfortable, remember that after you've recovered you can be the first one to drop off the casserole when someone else in your group needs help.

The woman was also creative in finding paid help. Insurance did not cover home health aides or homemakers for her, although she could do little for herself with two broken legs. Paying privately for such aides was prohibitively expensive. So she contacted a local college and hired students to come in to help her with tasks like washing her hair or putting in a load of laundry. It is possible to find mature people who can help you at a rate you can afford. They can use the extra money and flexible hours, and you can use the help.

Understand the burden of all this on your family. The patient said that sometimes her recovery was more emotionally difficult for her family than for her. When her mother flew in for two weeks to help, she arranged for her mother to stay at a friend's house so that it wasn't an around-the-clock chore for her. Her husband was supportive and helpful throughout, but at times it seemed he didn't grasp how the simplest tasks of daily living were out of her reach. It was impossible to maneuver her wheelchair through some of her doorways, and getting food was particularly difficult. The first day he had to go to work, he left her with a portable phone, an orange, and a pitcher of water. That wasn't going to feed her for the day and she had to tell her husband clearly what she needed and how he could help her have enough food within reach.

JUST IN CASE . . .

Advance Directives

No one relishes the idea of making preparations in case they become incapacitated or die. And it can feel especially uncomfortable to do it when you are about to go through a life event that has overtones of serious illness and mortality.

But it's important to state as clearly as you can what treatment you want if you ever get to a point when you can no longer speak for yourself. Such a statement, ideally in writing, is called an advance directive.

It's not that you need to dwell on horrible and unlikely events. But as new technologies are available that can keep you alive in a manner to which you are *not* accustomed, and in a way that you may have never contemplated, the question comes up: Do you want those procedures done on you? Increasingly people are answering that question by documenting what is acceptable and what is not acceptable treatment on their own bodies.

It can be done in several forms, by preparing a living will, designating a health-care proxy, and issuing a do-not-resuscitate order. These enable you to make sure the actions and decisions on your health will be *your* wishes, not someone else's preferences. If you just assume that your loved ones and helpers would naturally do what you want even if you're not able to say it yourself, consider the results of a recent study. In a waiting room, patients and the relatives accompanying them were asked the same four questions about what kind of care the patient would want. In almost all cases, the answers from the companions were different from those of the patients.

By making a written statement, you can help avoid divisive family disputes. Even though you're not conscious of the battles, would you want your brothers shouting about life and death as they gather around your comatose body? For some people, the process is too anxiety-producing and they simply don't believe in preparing a living will or designating a health-care proxy. If you fall in that category, do at least discuss the matter with your doctor.

If you're nineteen and you need an appendectomy, but are perfectly healthy otherwise, there isn't a great need to discuss issues like resuscitation in the aftermath of the surgery. But if you are sixty-five, have chronic heart failure and diabetes, and are about to undergo an appendectomy, it is sensible to have that conversation.

Your Doctor's Role

You might feel you're off the hook about this topic because your doctor never brought it up. Studies have shown that patients will say, "Sure, I've read about a living will and an agent who follows through on your wishes, but my doctor's never asked me, so I haven't done anything." If you see yourself as a consumer buying medical care, details like who brings up the topic first won't matter. You want to make your own choices.

If you haven't put instructions in writing, or even talked about it, doctors have different views about what to do if your medical condition critically worsens. Some may never recommend the removal of life support; others see it as the best option in a futile situation. Doctors dislike having to ask a patient's family to sign an instruction, like a do-not-resuscitate order. It places an enormous burden of guilt on a patient's family. As medical professionals, however, in matters of life and death, doctors should not abdicate their critical role as advisor.

In one extreme case a patient had a major stroke after surgery. He was comatose, on a respirator and artificial circulatory-support devices, and on dialysis for his failed kidneys. The surgeon recognized that continued treatments were prolonging death rather than prolonging life.

With no instruction from the patient in advance, the doctor went to the family and told them the physicians treating the patient had carefully discussed the matter and concluded that things had reached a state of medical futility. There was no realistic chance that the patient would recover. He said it was his recommendation at this point to turn off life-sustaining devices. The family agreed the doctor should continue to care for the patient, but without the aid of life-support systems.

Ethics Committee

Every hospital has an ethics committee or a legal advisor who reviews these issues. The committee will issue a recommendation based on the patient's file and discussion with the doctors, family members, and social workers. The physicians' input counts a great deal. The ethics committee will make sure that the patient is at the point where termination of life support is a legitimate question and seek the most clear and convincing evidence of what the patient would have wanted or whether continued treatment is truly futile.

The ethics committee is also called on to issue a recommendation when there is a dispute among family members. A written document such as a living will, even if it's been done in another state, holds a great deal of weight in such discussions. Verbal instructions also help, but are not as strong a piece of evidence as written instructions of a patient's wishes. The committee's intention is to help the family members gain perspective, find a common ground, and come to a consensus.

The Importance of Preparing Your Own Directives

All medical professionals have surprise—some might call them horror—stories. What to do when you have a patient in intensive care and find out he has two complete sets of wives and children who until now didn't know each other existed? Instead of being a provider of health care, the doctor ends up being the referee in a battle where people who love the patient hate each other. In this case, it was determined that the first wife was the legal one and had the right to decide the patient's care. But the resolution came after everyone went through a great deal of extra pain and confusion.

Although you probably aren't a bigamist, you have to recognize that you may reach the point of medical futility and *someone* has to make a decision about what to do next. Tell your doctor what you believe you would want done in such circumstances. Discuss it with your family. It's better to write it down, but if you can't, at least talk about it with the important people in your life. If you are the relative or friend of a person who is going to have surgery, have a frank discussion with that person and encourage him or her to make a living will and assign a health-care proxy.

Life, death, and medical intervention fuel passions that you may not have known existed among your relatives. For one man in a coma, even the doctor's belief that he would never come out of it and his wife's insistence that he surely did not want to live on life support was not enough for some relatives. When the feeding tubes were removed by the doctor at the wife's request, the relatives took the issue to court. The matter was resolved when the man died shortly thereafter.

As a patient you might not focus on the question of what happens if you're incapacitated—until you're in the hospital and surgery is imminent. Then you panic about the "what ifs" and start to dictate how to resolve some very difficult questions. Clearly, your mind is not at its sharpest and tension runs high; it is not an optimal time to make these decisions.

You might wonder what all this talk has to do with your surgery. You've already learned about the risks of your disease and the possible complications in surgery, and you feel confident that you will recover just fine. You don't even want to know about life-support systems and resuscitation orders in the extreme instances when a person needs them.

You also are aware that the worst-case scenario does sometimes happen. And not just after surgery. A person can be crossing the street when an eighteen-wheeler goes through a red light, and there he is—unconscious and heading for life support.

What would happen if the day after surgery you had a stroke or heart failure? What if you can't breathe on your own, your heart stops beating, but there's still life left in you? Who is the best person to decide which medical course among the available alternatives is the preferred one to follow? You are.

Ask yourself if you want doctors to do everything that's in the medical books to try to bring you back if you've stopped breathing. Or decide if you would rather have them stand aside and let nature take its course. Consider whether there are certain basic medical interventions that you do want performed, and others you don't. Recognize whether there is anyone else who really knows what you want and if that person has the authority from you to inform the doctors about it.

As you go through this process, understand that you do have the right to refuse or accept medical treatment, including life-sustaining treatment. You have the right to consent to treatment before it is started, and to have it stopped once it has begun. You can change your mind about what happens to you and about who you designate to speak on your behalf, even after you've put it in writing.

If making these choices in advance makes you feel uneasy, realize that if you've stated you don't want certain types of treatments, it doesn't mean that medical professionals will walk away from you and allow you to die. You will be maintained in comfort, and treatments not covered by your directives, such as fluids, tube feeding, pain medication, and drug therapy, will continue. Further, just because you have requested not to be maintained on life-support systems doesn't mean immediate end of life.

You are trying to cover extreme situations at any point in your life, including before and after surgery. For the duration of an operation, you are making an agreement with your doctor that he will perform surgery and do everything possible to get you through it. If you have any specific questions about what could happen during surgery and what steps should be taken to deal with problems in surgery, you can discuss those circumstances, which your doctor will document in your chart.

It is important to check with your doctor on the laws in your state that govern advance directives. The social-work and patient-relations staff in the hospital are very helpful resources. Or you can speak to a lawyer.

The following are some of the available options that can ensure your voice is heard, even if you can't speak at that moment.

Living will. This is a written document that expresses in advance your instructions and choices about various types of medical treatments and conditions. General instructions might not be very effective in carrying out your wishes, so try to be as specific as possible. For example, if you say you don't want "extreme measures," that may not be clear enough for a doctor to decide whether or not to use a treatment. But if you say: "I do not want to receive food and water through a tube if I am permanently unconscious with no hope of recovering," that is very clear. An example of a living will is included in Appendix B, pages 321–22.

Health-care agent. You can appoint someone over the age of eighteen whom you trust to act as your agent. That person, usually a close relative, can decide about your treatment if you lose the ability to decide for yourself. Consider to whom you would say in advance of a medical crisis, "These are my thoughts, this is how I feel. I am asking you to carry out the task of informing the doctor to do this for me. I trust you and I know you have the strength to do this for me."

You can write on the proxy form any information about treatment that you do or do not want. Your agent has to follow your instructions. You can also select an alternate agent if the one you've picked becomes unavailable or unwilling to make a decision. You can limit your agent's authority and either allow the designation to run indefinitely or put an expiration date or condition for its expiration on the form. Your agent is relied upon when doctors decide that you are not able to make health-care decisions for yourself.

Appendix C (pages 323–24) contains a sample health-care proxy statement. It is straightforward and does not require interpretation or the need for a lawyer. It does require two witnesses who are not the agents you are designating. This is the New York State form; you should find out what forms are acceptable in your state, as they do vary somewhat.

This type of designation is particularly important at a time when people are in nontraditional relationships. Your live-in companion for the last twenty years has no legal standing, but your mother whom you rarely see does. Put a great deal of thought into whom you would appoint. One woman, a medical professional who was used to dealing with difficult problems all day long, described the experience of being a health-care proxy for her mother as the hardest thing she ever had to do in her life.

Her mother had emphysema and pneumonia and when the doctor said she could only be kept alive on mechanical ventilation, the daughter said no. The doctor disagreed with the daughter, but she stood her ground. Her mother had polio as a child and was in an iron lung for a year. She stated that she absolutely did not want a life where she was immobile and could not breathe on her own. The daughter had to muster the strength to say to the doctor, "You don't understand. Your best outcome is my mother's worst nightmare."

When you choose a proxy, bear in mind that you are picking someone who may have to stand up to doctors and loved ones and say no.

Do-not-resuscitate order (DNR). Issued at your request, this is an instruction to the medical staff not to try to revive you through cardiopulmonary resuscitation (CPR) if your breathing or heartbeat has stopped. This request does not affect other types of treatments or procedures that can be done for you, such as antibiotics for an infection or use of a dialysis machine.

Without such an order, CPR will likely be applied to the fullest extent possible. This includes mouth-to-mouth resuscitation, external chest compression, electric shock, insertion of a tube to open your airway, injection of medication into your heart, or opening your chest to massage your heart.

You can also state that you would want some of these alternatives, but not all. You can agree to be subjected to external compression of the chest, for example, but not to an open-chest heart massage.

Why wouldn't a patient want CPR? Under most circumstances, people certainly would want to have everything done to keep them alive. But what if a patient is terminally ill or permanently unconscious and his heart stops? In that case, he may say in advance that he does not want to prolong life through resuscitation. It is sometimes medically clear that resuscitation will be futile or the expected outcome would leave a patient in a medical condition that is unacceptable to him. Some people feel they would rather not prolong the emotional and financial drain on their families if there is no hope that they will ever recover. In some cases, CPR may only partially succeed, leaving the patient brain-damaged or significantly impaired.

You probably have thought about some of these topics, at least in passing. Perhaps you've seen a news item about someone on life support and thought, "I don't ever want to end my days connected to tubes, living like a vegetable." Or maybe your beliefs about religion and science include the conviction that as long as technology has a way to sustain life, no man should be able to pull the plug on it.

What happened to the patient who discussed with her daughter that she absolutely did not want to be kept alive by any sort of feeding machine if it was clear that she wouldn't recover? She never arranged to designate her daughter as health-care proxy or put any of this in writing. Nor had she discussed her feelings with her doctor. Meanwhile, in the midst of the crisis, her son flew in from across the country. His mother's decision not to have feeding tubes was news to him. He was horrified by his sister's insistence that life support be removed. And the trauma of a mother's illness turned into a deeper struggle of how a family decides life-and-death issues.

Wills

If you haven't drawn up a will—and almost everyone has good reason to—it is helpful to do so as part of putting your house in order before surgery. However, it does not make sense to make a will if taking the time to prepare it would jeopardize the outcome of your surgery. If you are facing emergency surgery because of a ruptured aneurysm, that is not a time to redo your will.

The point of making a will in advance of surgery is not to delay an operation that needs to be done quickly or to become so emotionally distraught over preparing the terms of the will that you can't focus on what you need to do for the operation. It is to help you avoid making serious decisions when you are very ill, in pain, or distracted by medical issues.

If it seems far-fetched to consider a will in advance of surgery, medical professionals who are on the scene do not think so. They have seen it all, including the children who came to the hospital for their father to sign a will determining who would inherit his business, even as he was recovering from brain surgery in the intensive-care unit.

Notary publics, who can witness the signing of a will, are often on the staff of hospitals. They are usually specially trained to determine if a patient is signing a will freely, with full mental capacity, and without undue pressure from the family.

Power of Attorney

Mom has had a stroke and can't speak or write. Her rent has to be paid, her finances have to be handled—and you have no authority to do so. A family already distraught over illness becomes only more so as the business of life interjects itself. No one can just step in, cash mom's check, and pay her bills.

To prevent this from happening, you can prepare a power of attorney. This is a legal form that allows another person to sign your checks, deal with your finances, and tackle other practical matters. You can prepare a general power of attorney; also, check with your bank to see if they have a specific form they prefer you sign for your accounts at that bank. If you are helping someone who is going to have surgery, encourage that person to find out what a power of attorney can do for them and to decide whom they trust enough to empower.

A HEALTHY ATTITUDE

Some people won't need to read this section at all. A positive inner state comes naturally to them, no matter what is happening externally. Perhaps they've always been that way, or they've worked on themselves over the years to develop a way to face challenges without fear or anxiety.

At the other end of the spectrum is the patient who feels he is going to die in surgery. He may even feel at that moment that he wishes he could die. That can be a signal to a doctor to stop in his tracks, and postpone or even cancel surgery. No doctor wants to lose a patient in surgery, and if a patient is focused on dying rather than healing, then going through an operation at this time may have to be reconsidered. The doctor has to talk to the patient more about his feelings and refer him to psychological counseling.

For many people the diagnosis of an illness that is serious enough to require surgery is an emotional whack in the head. They feel their lives are out of control and they experience bouts of depression and anger. The patient, his close family, and friends go through a difficult emotional time. The whole process can lead to a tailspin of fear and negative thinking.

It doesn't have to. There are ways to restore positive thinking and feelings of control that may have dissipated during diagnosis and decision making.

First, talk about it. Get your feelings aired and acknowledged. Often, you need a way to ventilate those feelings outside the family system. Although family and friends may be enormously supportive, at times they too show the strains of your illness and can express anger when what you need is comfort. You may feel your family members sometimes approach you with the attitude of "How dare you get sick. You're ruining my life." Or they'll try to take control, showing their exasperation by saying things like, "It's as obvious as the nose on your face you have to have surgery. So don't sit around and cry about it. Snap out of it and get going." People use many ways to detach from the emotional pain, including ones that make the pain sharper.

For both you and your family, just being able to go to a place where you feel safe, and are free to say what you want, can be very therapeutic. It can lift some of the anxiety and depression that comes from repressing strong feelings.

Recognize that even when there's every reason to expect to recover fully from your disease, at the time you absorb the initial impact of the news, it sometimes feels like you'll never get over it. It is natural to feel anxiety about the unknown. Any diagnosis that impacts your daily experience, even for a short period, is life-changing. When it's a serious matter that threatens the fabric of your life, or your survival, you may go through stages of grief similar to the loss of a loved one. That includes a period of denial, a time to be openly sad, and a time to move on and cope with the realities. Part of the grieving process is feeling anger that this is happening to you. You never smoked, you exercised—and you still had a heart attack. A normal response to that sense of injustice is, "Why me?"

Restoring hope and feeling positive, so that you can undergo the surgery and heal, can be hard work. You may already have a network—a therapist, a religious counselor, a support group, or a family structure that you can turn to for help.

Many people also look to resources available through their doctor's office and the hospital. Doctors are likely to know of support groups made up of people who have the same illness you have and have already gone through the operation you are facing. They can also refer you to the therapists on staff in the social-work department of the hospital. These counselors are particularly skilled in knowing how to listen actively to patients and respond to their needs with the sensitivity and respect that is appropriate to someone coping with a health problem.

Sometimes people prefer to speak with a religious counselor. They may want someone with whom to pray or they may be experiencing a crisis that is not only physical and emotional, but also spiritual. They need to express feelings like, "Is God really there? How could He let this happen to me?" If a patient is away from home or doesn't have a person to call on, most hospitals have a pastoral services unit that matches patients with ministers, priests, and rabbis who regularly work with the hospital.

For others, their desire to develop a positive attitude through a time of medical challenge is helped by the techniques of complementary medicine. Meditation brings a feeling of calm; visualization and guided imagery can help a person imagine his disease leaving his body. If people are in pain, they may seek out acupuncture. If they are stressed out at points in the day, a cup of soothing herbal tea or a series of yoga postures may restore equilibrium. For others, audiotapes that use tonal music and affirmation can help induce relaxation.

Find out what works for you. Your goal is clear: replace fear and anxiety with positive thoughts and a feeling of calm, so that your surgery and recovery will be aided by your own inner healing resources.

If you are feeling any stress from your diagnosis and impending treatment, don't ignore it. The stress response isn't just a thing of the mind. It can lead to physical changes like a decrease in blood supply to parts of your body, less clarity in your thinking, increased blood pressure, and shallow breathing. A weakened body and a distracted mind can lower your resistance and prolong your recovery. The sweaty palms you feel are just one visible manifestation of stress; internally there can be a lot of changes that can make it harder for your body to cope.

All these matters—what you should eat, how you delegate your work, who can make health-care decisions on your behalf, and where to express your emotions—are ancillary to the operation itself. You could check into the hospital, have your surgery, and leave without ever tackling any of these questions head on. But then you're leaving yourself open to some major aftershocks.

For most patients, an operation is not an event in isolation. They usually realize that they have to change some part of their lifestyle, confront the fact that mortality is a reality, and deal with the emotional issues raised by such stress. You can't turn your life around in the weeks before surgery, and you probably don't need to. But as you prepare for your operation, you can ensure that it is the best physical and psychological experience that it can be. Take care of your body's extra needs, assign your responsibilities to others, prepare directives that keep your wishes paramount, and be open to receiving support to get through what, by any measure, is a tough time.

These are tasks for you to do while still at home. In the next chapter, I will explore in greater detail how you can use the hospital to its fullest extent. It is not just the arena for your top-notch medical team to do its work. It's also a repository of special services to help you get through the medical process with the least difficulty. Who are you likely to find there, and why and how should you use their services?

6

Using Special Services

A hospital is no hotel when it comes to luxury and relaxation. But if you or a loved one is having surgery, where else can you line up the services you'll need to donate blood, find a quality nursing home for an ailing parent, and arrange to get the TV hooked up?

Hospitals are geared to work out patients' problems, from the most complicated treatments to the most mundane logistics. However, people are typically in the hospital for such a short time now, so the fact that there is so much available can get lost in the shuffle. Don't let it. A hospital maintains programs because thousands of other patients in your situation have been there, done that—and needed those services.

Thumb through those glossy brochures in earnest and learn just what special services there are in the hospital and what they can do for you. Find out what won't cost you a penny more—visits from social workers for inpatients—and which items, like renting a TV, will be an extra charge.

Support services are one clear indication whether that institution sees you as a whole person, and treats you that way. Of course no listing in a brochure can adequately tell you whether the individuals providing that service will care for you in a way that brightens your spirit and comforts your body. Will a nurse's aide come in with a smile, fluff your pillow, and ask with sincerity, "How are you doing today?" That kind of information is more likely to come to you from other people's experiences as patients.

PATIENT RELATIONS

Has an aide been especially rude to you? Did a visitor leave her cassette player in your room, only to have it go missing? Is the patient in the bed next to you so noisy you can't get any sleep? You don't have to gnash your teeth and curse health-care institutions. You can call patient relations.

Traditionally known as an advocate for patients, this department in some hospitals is also called customer relations. Make no mistake about it. You may be attached to tubes, in pain, and barely able to move, but you are still a paying customer and if you have a complaint or a request, there is someone to act on it.

Patient relations can explain hospital procedures to you or track down the person who turns on phone service or find out why you got a different lunch from what you ordered. Sometimes a "courtesy visitor" from the department may pop into your room and say, "How's everything going? Is there anything you'd like us to know?" Use the opportunity to let the administration know your input about the day-to-day experiences of being a patient in that hospital.

The members of a patient-relations department are skilled in interpreting the hospital's policies and procedures, and in finding out what to do if they aren't being followed. They can help you with special requests and serve as a go-between with the medical personnel who are treating—or perhaps mistreating—you.

Food becomes a big issue for many patients, and a big source of complaint. Now that you're in the hospital, the low-salt, low-fat diet you're supposed to be on is a reality. You can't just run to the refrigerator and cheat. You eye the tray and say, "I don't like this low-fat salad dressing. I won't eat margarine." Patient relations can step in, speak to the appropriate department, and let them know you're having trouble eating. Maybe you'll need a staff person to explain your diet; maybe the kitchen is sending you the wrong tray. A good patient-relations department will investigate something as basic as your lunch and follow up by sending a representative to make sure your complaints have been addressed.

One of the department's jobs is to make sure you, and everyone who stays in the hospital, works in it, or visits it knows exactly what the rights of a patient are. "A Patient's Bill of Rights," which is mandated by the federal commission that accredits hospitals, is posted by patient relations in highly visible areas. Are your relatives cooling their heels by the elevator? They too can read about your rights before the door opens. It might come in handy.

The wording varies by state, but here are some of the specifics:

- Receive treatment without discrimination, including source of payment.

- Receive considerate and respectful care.

- Be in a clean, safe environment.

- Receive emergency care if you need it.

- Be informed of the name and position of the doctor who will be in charge of your care.

- Be informed of the names, positions, and functions of any hospital staff involved in your care.

- Be able to refuse treatment, examination, or observation by any of the hospital staff.

- Receive complete information about your diagnosis, treatment, and prognosis.

- Receive all the information you need—including risks and benefits—for any proposed procedure before you sign an informed consent.

- Receive all the information you need to make an order not to resuscitate or to designate a person to make that order for you.

- Be able to refuse treatment and be told what effects this may have on you.

- Be able to refuse to take part in research.

- Have privacy and confidentiality maintained for all your information and records.

- Participate in all decisions about treatment and discharge.

- Be provided with a written discharge plan and how you can appeal it.

- Review your medical record without charge.

- Obtain a copy of your medical record for a reasonable fee.

- Receive an itemized bill and explanation of all charges.

- Complain without fear of reprisals about care and services. Receive a response to complaints from the hospital. If you are not satisfied, be provided with the number of the state agency to file a complaint.

- Authorize which family members will be given priority to visit.

- Be able to document your wishes if you want to donate body parts.

- If there is anything you don't understand about these rights, the hospital must provide help, including a translator, so you can understand them.

Even if you don't remember all of the Patient's Rights, keep the spirit of them close to your heart. You have very broad and basic rights while you are in a hospital, and if you feel they are being violated, speak up. If you are a family member or a friend of a patient, be aware of those rights so that if you have to act as an advocate on behalf of someone who is too ill to speak for himself, you have the confidence to do that.

SOCIAL-WORK DEPARTMENT

Having an operation may well provoke a crisis in your life—medical, emotional, spiritual, financial, or all of these. Does your hospitalization feel like an overwhelming burden to you? Are you wondering how you will ever get help when you get out? Would you like to find other people who've had your surgery and talk to them?

Those are just a few of the issues that social workers who are employed by a hospital are skilled in handling. They can talk to you with the trained ears of a person who can help you during times of crises. They are essential to your discharge planning. And they can find support for you, whether it's through individual counseling or group discussion.

Hospital social workers help you as soon as you need them, a process called crisis intervention. Sometimes that intervention means talking to a patient who's flooded with feelings and helping him process what's happening to him. Or it may be a case of immediately directing a family on appropriate steps should an unforeseen complication occur as a patient is emerging from surgery and is unable to speak.

Depending on the size of the hospital and how it's structured, the social-work unit may be part of the different medical teams or may be assigned to a hospital floor. It may be called integrated care, case management, or discharge planning. A staff member from the department may go on rounds with the health-care team and screen patients' charts to identify what issues could come up. Using the help of social services is completely voluntary.

There are very good reasons to meet with the social-work staff before you are admitted to the hospital. Managed-care companies are not paying hospitals to keep you or your relative there while you work out which nursing home your father will go on to or what agency will supply you with a home health aide. Discharge planning starts not when you're about to leave, but before you arrive. The process can be very time-consuming and in order to have services arranged for you at the time you are medically ready, you need to begin early.

Before you arrive at the hospital, think about your life after surgery. Will you be able to shop, prepare meals, bathe, go to the bank, and get to doctor's appointments by yourself? Or will you need help for some of those activities, and for how long?

Social workers connect patients with agencies that supply visiting nurses and home health aides. They help patients sort out who's going to pay for those services. And if the patient can't go right back home, they work with the family to provide placement, such as referral to rehabilitation facilities or nursing homes.

You don't have to deal with the demanding issues by yourself, nor does your family. Every patient who comes to the hospital doesn't have to reinvent the wheel when it comes to what care he needs, what agency will provide it, and where to find it. There are experienced people who can navigate the system and make recommendations to you.

Sometimes the needs are simply logistical. For example, where can your family stay while you're in the hospital so that it won't cost more than your entire surgery bill? Often, especially in large cities, hospitals make arrangements with local hotels to provide rooms at a discounted rate. There may even be shuttle service to bring families back and forth. Some hospitals also have specially funded housing or apartments for patients and families when longer-term treatment is necessary. You can't know all of this, but you can expect a social-work department to know it. Ask any question that's on your mind.

If you've never used a social-work staff before, this is the time to find out if there's something you haven't thought of, that could make a difference. Sometimes you are worried about a family member or a job issue that you would rather not discuss with your surgeon, but you would feel comfortable raising with a social worker. Chances are, you or your family members could use an experienced shoulder to lean on when you need to express some of the powerful feelings that often accompany illness and surgery.

A patient's biggest concern besides the surgery itself is money. Who is going to pay for everything? Social workers are not insurance people, but they can educate you about Medicaid, Medicare, and private insurance. And they can tell you where to go for more information. Social workers can help you figure out how to resolve problems and point you toward policy and case managers and billing departments.

If you are an inpatient, you do not have to pay an additional amount to receive help from the social-services department in the hospital, just as you don't pay extra for nurses. Of course, those costs are bundled into basic hospital charges, so whether you use them or not, you've contributed to the kitty. Outpatients may be billed if they use hospital social workers; this charge is usually covered by insurance, but as in all matters of insurance, you have to check.

COMPLEMENTARY MEDICINE

Do you think hypnosis means you'll be made to bark like a dog and cluck like a chicken? That yoga requires shaving your head, dressing in orange, and chanting? Not true. Techniques like hypnosis and yoga are cropping up even in the most conservative hospital environments, and for very good reason. They can help you relax, fight off depression, and create an optimum environment for healing.

You still won't find these complementary medicine departments, as they're called, at every hospital. Many patients have to look to resources outside the hospital system to find out about the techniques. As the number of people using these therapies grows, physicians are becoming increasingly aware of them. At the very least, a responsible medical professional wants to know whether his patients are taking megavitamins, using herbal medicines, or practicing another unconventional technique in addition to what he is prescribing.

Studies of patients who have had surgery at Columbia-Presbyterian show that 70 percent of them use some form of complementary-medicine technique. Pioneering research in the validity of these techniques is being done through the Department of Complementary Medicine Services at the hospital. The department offers patients the opportunity to use mind-body techniques, often referred to as modalities, in partnership with the treatments of conventional Western medicine, known as allopathic medicine.

The aim of using these techniques when undergoing surgery is to short-circuit the stress response, a reaction that generally makes you feel awful and probably impairs your healing process. You decrease pain, stress, and anxiety through finding a technique that is comfortable for you.

Complementary medicine is not a magic bullet. It is a tool that empowers a patient in the medical process. It's not for someone who figures, "The doctor will fix me, I'll go home, and go back to being a couch potato and eat a zillion potato chips." Rather, complementary-medicine techniques are something you have to contribute to, while believing the benefits are worth the effort it takes.

In hospitals, these techniques are used as an adjunct to traditional medicine, not as a replacement. For example, if you have lower back problems, you still pursue the best approach to alleviating the symptoms through medication, physical therapy, or surgery, but you also learn meditation or yoga to help you deal with the pain.

Representative options available through Columbia-Presbyterian's Complementary Medicine Department include the following:

- **Audiotapes.** Specially designed to help encourage relaxation and a smoother return to awareness after anesthesia, these are made up of scientifically researched sounds called binaural beats, which balance the right and left sides of the brain. They are embedded at a very low volume and are the background for music and voices that evoke serene and positive images. Patients listen to the tapes prior to surgery, during surgery while under anesthesia, and in the recovery room.

- **Hypnosis.** Also called hypnotherapy, hypnosis is a technique to induce a very relaxed state of focused concentration. You do not lose control of your actions nor are you manipulated. Hypnosis is a voluntary process. The intention is to create a sense of relaxation so deep that you can help control pain and create a sense of well-being. A hypnotherapist uses words that evoke peaceful, soothing scenarios to engage a patient's imagination and help him enter a trancelike state where he is alert, but relaxed. You can also enter this free-floating feeling by using tapes or learning to do self-hypnosis.

- **Guided imagery.** Using the power of the mind to evoke a physical response, you can learn how to use images through audiotapes, in group classes, or in private sessions with a practitioner. There is no single standard way to approach guided imagery. Practitioners may become certified at any one of a number of institutes or training academies around the country, which are often run by psychologists. Further, guided imagery in hospital settings is done by professionals who have not only been trained in the techniques, but who have a couple of years of clinical experience in a medical specialty like nursing. The idea behind guided imagery is to learn how to use mental images to reduce stress, slow heart rate, stimulate the immune system, and reduce pain.

- **Reflexology.** This involves pressure applied to specific areas of the hands and feet, which can benefit other points of the body. It is sometimes used in intensive care or immediately after surgery.

- **Acupressure.** Based on European healing practices, it balances the flow of life energy in the body. Practitioners apply gentle but firm finger pressure to points identified throughout the body. This technique is often used pre-operatively and during recovery. These massage techniques are intended to induce a relaxed but aware state, helping to heal while improving circulation and encouraging a sense of physical and emotional well-being.

- **Yoga.** Ancient practices derived from Hinduism to try to unify the mind and body include stretching, breathing, and meditative positions or postures. They strengthen the body and create balance and peace of mind.

- **Qigong/tai chi.** These are ancient Chinese exercises for stimulating and balancing *qi,* or vital life energy. They are gentle physical movements done with a calm mind and regular breaths to encourage the circulation of *qi* in the body. Some claim this technique is effective in improving the immune and digestive systems, reducing pain and insomnia, and lowering blood pressure.

Other therapies that you may hear about and want to investigate for help in the surgical process include acupuncture (fine needles inserted into special points in the body), consulting with an herbalist to learn which herbs to take, and using vitamins and foods as a boost to healing. As with anything you take by mouth or do with your body, find out what the risks are and the benefits. Do not assume because a doctor doesn't have to write out a prescription for an herb or megavitamin that it isn't potent. Make sure your doctor approves any herbal supplement or megavitamin you plan to take.

If all this seems too unfamiliar and somewhat suspect, you may want no part of it. It may cause you stress rather than relieve it. But if you have an open mind, or if you're already familiar with mind-body treatments, consider whether it can help you now as you have surgery. You'll need to find a match with a treatment that is right for you. About five to ten days before surgery is a good time to start one of these techniques. And you may want to continue well after you go home so that whatever benefits you got in the hospital will continue to help you stay on a health and wellness path.

These services are not standard fare yet, and they are generally not currently covered by insurance. You will have to pay out-of-pocket if you want to learn guided imagery or purchase tapes for the operating room.

The body of knowledge is growing, however, and as studies using accepted scientific methods convincingly associate these techniques with improved health, attitudes—and insurance coverage—regarding complementary medicine have begun to change.

BLOOD-DONOR SERVICES

Another common source of anxiety for many people is that they might need a blood transfusion and that the blood will be somehow contaminated with the virus that causes AIDS or another disease.

Instead of worrying, give blood—your own or that of your relatives. If you're well enough, you can donate your own blood, called an *autologous blood donation.* There is clearly a reduction in the risk of infection and allergic reaction if you use your own blood. Your doctor will determine how much you need and set up a schedule for giving blood and having it set aside for you, which usually takes place at the hospital where you are having surgery. Typically these appointments run about a week apart until enough blood is collected. If you want to do this, be sure you request it well enough in advance of surgery so you can provide the amount of blood you need over a reasonable period of time. It's likely that you may have to take iron pills for about a month. A bonus is that if you don't need the blood, it will be kept for someone else's use.

If you can't give your own blood, you might think that the next best thing is to arrange for a relative or friend to donate blood for you. That is a misconception, however. Having a relative or friend give blood for you is no safer than getting blood from a blood bank. In reality, the incidence of diseases like hepatitis and of allergic reactions is no greater from a general blood bank than it is from designated donors.

Although relatives are encouraged to donate blood to a blood bank, hospitals discourage them from donating blood for a specific individual. If you insist on having blood donated by a relative for your surgery, many hospitals will allow it, but at an extra cost that's charged directly to the patient or the donor. Such blood can't be put with the general blood supply. It has to be specially tagged and brought to the operating room for the patient. If you donate your own blood, you do not have to pay extra.

The idea of using blood from someone a patient knows cropped up as a response to fears about HIV, the virus that causes AIDS. The ability to screen the blood supply for HIV is so good now, however, that getting blood from a relative does not add to the safety of the blood you are getting. Instead of succumbing to fears about blood and relying on a directed donation that has no proven benefit, arrange to donate your own blood or assure yourself about the safety of the general blood supply.

PRIVATE-DUTY NURSING

Do visions of horror run across your mind as you see yourself lying helpless in your hospital bed? Need something desperately, but can't reach the buzzer? You reach the buzzer, but still no one comes?

You can hire a private-duty nurse, someone who is there just for you, at your bedside, responding to your needs, checking on your vital signs. The catch is you have to pay for it. For many people, a private-duty nurse is a necessary luxury in the hours immediately after surgery, but not for an extended period of time.

Technically, no one in a hospital needs a private-duty nurse. If you are in a risky situation where you require a close watch, you'll be in an intensive-care unit. If you're stable, you'll be on a hospital floor where the regular nurses and aides care for you.

That doesn't mean you won't want your own nurse. If the patient down the hall needs CPR and you need a glass of water, the nursing staff will be in that other patient's room and you'll have to wait. For some people, that extra care and attention is available by having family members stay for long hours at the hospital. These days, hospitals are generally far more open to the presence of a husband or a daughter who stays past visiting hours to cater to a patient's needs.

If you don't have a family member available and it's important to you to have someone at your side, and you can afford it, the hospital should provide you with the telephone number for the registry of private-duty nurses. These nurses are not employed by the hospital, but by you. A hospital won't let just any nurse work on its premises, so the registry is composed of nurses who have been approved to care for patients on site.

Since a private-duty nurse works on a shift basis, with a shift usually lasting either eight or twelve hours, patients can opt for the service for the period of time when they most need constant care. Furthermore, there are different skill levels of nursing available— registered nurse, licensed practical nurse, or nurse's aide—and the hourly rate is priced accordingly. You can discuss with your doctor what level of nursing care you're likely to need after surgery.

Thanks to newer procedures, patients often come out of major surgery in much better shape than they used to. For example, almost everyone who had open-heart surgery used to hire a private-duty nurse. Now it's rare.

Nevertheless, you may well want to have a skilled professional who is there for you in the hours or days after surgery, and your hospital should make it easy for you to hire that person. It is generally up to you, or your relatives, to make the request and follow through on the arrangements.

CHAPLAIN'S SERVICES

There is no reason to forego the comfort of spiritual support just because you are at a distance from home, or don't have easy access to a religious counselor. Hospitals are able to provide the services of a priest, minister, or rabbi, at your bedside, at your request.

Not all denominations are represented. For example, you may not be able to find an Islamic cleric through the chaplain's office, which is also called pastoral services. But you can ask whether there is another option available. For example, in medical centers where there is a Muslim population, employees of the center may have a prayer group available to visit with Muslim patients and pray with them.

Religious counselors are not usually on the staff of a hospital, but are on call, sometimes twenty-four hours a day. For the most part, representatives of the major religious faiths are available for counseling and prayer; performance of services would be limited to what can be reasonably done at the bedside. There may also be nondenominational counselors who can provide support outside the context of a specific religious practice.

Many hospitals also have chapels that can be used for quiet prayer or meditation; often religious services are performed there. Ask for a schedule if one hasn't already been provided. If your doctor says you are well enough to go, you will be escorted to and from a service, and you can wear your hospital gown.

TRANSLATION DEPARTMENT

Concerned that your relative is having surgery and doesn't speak English? A cadre of translators who speak several different languages are on call to translate, especially in larger metropolitan areas. Sign-language interpreters are also likely to be available.

It may happen that the patient speaks English well enough, but the family doesn't, and they need help to talk to the medical staff. No reasonable request to provide a translator will be refused, if a person speaking that language is available. But a hospital doesn't hire translators as part of its staff. Rather, translators either work on a voluntary basis from the community, or are staff members who are fluent in a language and have agreed to be called on to translate.

In an area where a hospital serves a large population of people who speak another language, basic information should be available in that language as well as English. For example, many hospital brochures and instructions are now also printed in Spanish.

OTHER SERVICES

There are many other services you should expect a quality hospital to offer. They may not be essential to your surgery, but they help make the experience for you, your family, and your friends as tolerable as possible. These include:

- Automatic teller machines.

- Beauty and barbershop facilities.

- Dining areas.

- Gift and flower shop.

- Guest services like parking and waiting rooms.

- Mail service.

- Reading materials.

- Television and video rentals.

- Telephone service.

A caring institution can go a long way toward making your hospital stay as positive and conducive to healing as possible. For the vast majority of patients today, the day they arrive at the hospital is the day they have surgery. In a well-run institution, there should be no obstacles that add tension and confusion to the process of arriving and being routed to surgery.

Throughout the process, you should feel a considerate response that instills faith in that medical care center. You aren't paying for a vacation, but you and your insurance company are paying for a place of rest and recuperation whose services are linked to your health and well-being in a far more serious way. You should be treated with the respect that any welcome guest is entitled to feel, and more so.

The next chapter addresses how to make that process work best for you, from first scheduling the operation, to undergoing anesthesia at the hospital.

7

Planning Your Hospitalization

It may be hard not to feel like a victim when you're about to have an operation. A heightened sense that you're losing some control over your short-term plans, and perhaps your long-term destiny, is unnerving. First you feel threatened by the disease or injury. Then you feel further demoralized by facing what appears to be the indignity of hospitalization. You see yourself eking out privacy in your room behind the thinnest of curtains. Clothed in a gown that barely covers your body, you feel vulnerable to medical personnel who are essentially strangers peering at you and prodding you at every turn. You've got to contend with insurance policies that dictate what medical care you can have and hospital policies that give you specific rules, like when you can have visitors.

It's enough to make you check out before you even check in. Instead, take a look at the process. Remember, it won't last long. Hospital stays today are shorter than ever. What can you do to make the experience better?

Surgery might be at the opposite end of the pleasure spectrum from a vacation, but when it comes to making plans, it's a valid comparison. To have as good an experience as possible, it's not enough just to say you're going to Paris. You have to schedule a hotel room, arrange transportation, and plan your activities.

Even in the best of circumstances, you can't control everything. It might rain for a week and the taxi drivers could go on strike. No one avoids all the vagaries of life, but if you make plans you're more likely to get what you want, like tickets to the opera or a convenient time to fly home.

Once you've decided that surgery is the best option for you, start taking the steps to make the entire process work in your best interest. Do the groundwork. As if you were planning for a trip or other major event, read the booklets and brochures about the hospital, go to its Web sites, talk to the nurses and staff in your doctor's office about what to expect, and schedule your surgery in a way that is as smooth and conducive to healing as possible.

Recognize that you do have a say in what is going to happen, even in routine matters. Find out what the options are and what choices are yours to make. Take any steps you can before you're in the hospital and before your energy is focused on recovering from surgery. The beginning of the process is a good time to plan the end of it. Put in motion your discharge arrangements. Think about whether you'll be able to prepare a meal and get to a doctor's appointment on your own, if you'll need to have a family member available, or whether you will have to hire someone.

Whatever aspect of your surgical experience that you're planning, get help wherever and whenever you need it. Ask your support group of family and friends to pitch in.

Let people know you're happy to have visitors. It is likely they will distract you, encourage you, and help you with information. The doctor stopped in and you can't remember what she just said? Your visitor, who isn't taking pain medication and is a lot more clearheaded at the moment, may well recall the doctor's comments. Visitors also keep you connected to the rest of your life at a time when you're disoriented.

Take advantage of the hospital's special services discussed in detail in Chapter 6. You are not bothering anyone by making such requests. Special services like chaplains to comfort you and social workers to plan your discharge are in the hospital to help you.

And give yourself a boost and a pat on the back whenever you need it. You are, after all, undergoing surgery to make your life better than it could be otherwise. Positive thinking goes a long way toward turning what may seem like an intolerable situation into an acceptable one.

The woman who had an abscess surgically removed from her labia got through the pain by reminding herself that she was not dealing with a cancerous tumor. For the patient who had a second surgery to remove the pins from both her legs broken in an accident two years earlier, it was comforting to know this time she could plan her surgery to coincide with the slow time in her business. The prospect of resting after the operation buoyed her spirits. And the man who had back surgery? The operation is now a blip on his radar screen. But the lifestyle he's resumed, including jogging and competing in triathlons, is an ongoing reality.

Try to remain positive so you can focus your energy on healing. What enables you to do something you dread? Do you tell yourself that it could be worse or that you're preventing more serious problems later? Or once this is over, you'll get back to doing the things you really love? It's not easy, but this is not likely the first time in your life you've had to give yourself a pep talk.

After you've talked to your doctor about having surgery, she won't just send you out to fend for yourself. She will set you up with her nurse, or other staff member, to make arrangements with the hospital. This is your opportunity to sit down one-on-one with a medical professional who will help you set surgery in motion by clearly discussing matters that include the following: scheduling appointments for surgery, pre-surgical testing, and anesthesia evaluation; getting the green light from insurance; understanding instructions for the hours before surgery and the check-in procedure.

MAKING ARRANGEMENTS

Scheduling an Appointment for Surgery

One of your first tasks is to set a date for surgery. A staff member in your doctor's office will act as an intermediary, usually while you are present, and call the hospital's admitting office to schedule a time.

What if you learn your surgeon is free and there's a bed available on a date that's immediately before your niece's wedding? The victim in you sighs and schedules the surgery for the first opportunity that's offered to you. The consumer in you recognizes that the first offer of any service does not have to be the last. Maybe you hate weddings and couldn't care less if you miss this one. Or maybe she's your favorite niece, you haven't seen your brother in a year, and it would really depress you to miss this family event. Instead of shrugging off your needs, question whether there are any medical risks in waiting a little longer. Find out if another day can reasonably be selected, one that lets you go to the wedding and have your operation in a timely manner.

There are always several factors to consider in scheduling an appointment. These include medical necessity, the surgeon's schedule, your personal plans, and the availability of beds. You may have to work out a compromise among conflicting demands, but your own priorities are equally relevant.

Arranging for a Room

There isn't usually much choice here, unless you can pay independently for a private room, a cost that may run an additional couple of hundred dollars per day over the amount that insurance will reimburse. Assigned to you by the hospital staff, your room will most likely be a double room shared with another patient. If an infection or other medical consideration requires you to be separate from other patients you will be placed in a single room. If it's a medical necessity, this should be covered by your health insurance. Another exception to being in the standard double room is in the case where you require constant supervision and are placed in an intensive-care unit for a period of time that extends from the time immediately after surgery to several weeks.

If there are problems with your room once you are in it, tell the appropriate people you need it fixed. You don't have to stay in a room that's dirty, unventilated, or lacking a piece of equipment. If the staff that is caring for you doesn't respond to your request for repair, ask a family member to speak to the patient-relations department, or do it yourself if you can. One of the tasks of patient relations is to handle such problems.

Lining Up Service

When you are scheduling your surgery, you can also schedule some of the special services you want, like arranging to have your own blood donated for your operation, using complementary-medicine techniques to help in healing, or contacting private-duty nurses.

If your family needs hotel accommodations, find out from your doctor's office if the hospital has any arrangements with local hotels to provide rooms at special rates to patients' families. Book early, as the supply of such rooms may be limited. If you need special transportation to the hospital, find out what is available, how much it costs, who makes the arrangements, and how much advance notice you need.

Contacting Medical Insurers

The issue of who is going to pay is a major concern for anyone who is undergoing an operation. The surgeon's staff can arrange to get routine approval from your insurance company by calling them and supplying them with the information they need. The doctor's office will then forward information on your medical insurance coverage to the hospital's admitting and billing departments.

It doesn't always go smoothly, however. In any given situation, you can't always know what to expect from your health insurance company. For patients facing an operation, it can sometimes feel like the rules are being made up as they go along. At the very least, you're likely to have many questions. Are you covered under a government-sponsored plan like Medicare or Medicaid and what does that mean for your choices? Is the surgeon you want in your HMO network? If you have traditional insurance that lets you go to whatever doctor and hospital you want, how much is your copayment?

Your surgeon's office should be equipped with staff who are knowledgeable and willing to help you sort through this from the start. And at the finish, you should have a clear idea of who is paying and for what, as well as an authorization number or other form of verification from your insurer that you can bring with you to the admitting office on the day of surgery.

In between those points, you may have to work out some tough issues. This may be your first pass at dealing with medical insurance beyond a routine examination or having a prescription filled at a pharmacy. Even if you choose not to get a second opinion, your insurance company may require one for approval. Your surgeon may do the operation on an inpatient basis; your insurance will only reimburse that type of surgery on an outpatient basis. You need a certain type of operation and no surgeon in your plan does it. This creates the need to negotiate with your insurer who may be either strict about its policies or lenient in bending them for you.

Learn the details of your plan. Speak to your insurer directly. And request that the staff in your surgeon's office be your ally in working your way through the insurance process. The benefits department of your employer will also help you negotiate with your insurance company. They are a good resource and are likely to get answers for you much more expeditiously.

Pre-surgical Testing

Pre-surgical testing is essential to schedule in advance of surgery. This includes lab tests and an examination by an internist, and it is generally done between one week and one month before your operation—unless of course your surgery is an emergency.

These tests are done to make sure you're physically fit to have surgery. They establish a baseline reading of your medical status and identify any problems that need to be evaluated and possibly treated before an operation takes place.

For example, a patient in his fifties came in for pre-surgical testing for orthopedic surgery. The examination found that his blood pressure was elevated. If it stayed too high, he couldn't have the surgery. So the internist started medication to lower his blood pressure in advance of surgery. The patient had to come back again to assure the treatment was effective and the surgery could be done on schedule. Even once he was cleared for surgery, he was checked again on the morning of surgery.

The examining doctor does not ignore the role of a health risk like high blood pressure in your long-term picture. But she will refer you to someone else, like your own internist, for evaluation and treatment who will focus on keeping your blood pressure under control so that it is optimal for surgery.

Although some pre-surgical tests are necessary, you don't need to have all of them. This will depend on the type of surgery you are having and your own health. Any time that you are tested, whether it's for surgery or another matter, question what tests are being done and why.

The major reasons for pre-surgical testing are to verify the state of your health, identify any problems that could make a difference in the operation, and help identify the most effective and safest method of anesthesia for you. When you are admitted on the day of surgery, you won't need to go through another round of tests, unless there is some reason such as the appearance of a new symptom or a recheck of an old one.

Pre-surgical testing is done based on the following: age, pre-existing medical conditions, and type of surgery. If you are older than forty, in general you need a greater range of tests as a matter of course, such as a chest X ray or an EKG (electrocardiogram). If you are thirty, you should expect to have only blood tests. Regardless of your age, if the surgery is more complicated or if you have other health problems, the doctor will order more extensive tests.

You can have the testing and exam done where it is most convenient for you. Generally, it is done at the medical center where you will have your surgery. The results can be immediately entered into the system and made available to the doctors who will be treating you in the course of surgery. If you are traveling a distance for the surgery or if you have a complicated medical problem that requires close supervision by your doctor, you may have your testing done by your own internist. In that case, the results will be sent to the medical center and entered in your file.

At the time of the testing, an internist will examine you, check your blood pressure, find out what medications you're taking, and determine if any tests other than those ordered by your surgeon need to be done.

The basic tests include:

- *Blood tests.* A blood sample will be collected, most often just for blood count and chemistry. In special circumstances, such as a big operation, the blood test will also be used to test how long it takes your blood to clot. If you have any problem with clotting, the doctors do not want to wait until you are being operated on to find out. You could hemorrhage large amounts of blood. Blood tests are also done to determine your body's chemistry, for example, the levels of blood sugar and potassium, and to make sure the liver and kidneys are functioning normally. A blood count is taken to make sure you are not anemic.

- *Urine test.* A urinalysis is done to make sure you don't have a urinary-tract infection, especially if you are having the type of surgery where an infection could easily spread. The urine is also checked to see if there are any abnormalities in it like sugar or blood.

- *Chest X ray.* This is done to find out if there is a malignancy, emphysema, or the presence of anything, like an infection, in the lungs that could cause shortness of breath, make anesthesia more difficult, or delay your recovery.

- *Electrocardiogram (EKG).* There are certain types of irregularities that a doctor can detect in an EKG that would indicate an increased risk of problems during surgery, like an irregular heartbeat or a previous heart attack.

The results of the tests take about a day. If all the tests are normal, you get clearance from the internist who does the review. The internist writes a note that you are medically stable for surgery and puts that on your chart. If the test results do not directly affect your surgery, like the presence of a higher than normal cholesterol level, then the internist may recommend that you work on your cholesterol, but she would not delay surgery.

If something shows up in the tests and exam that the internist sees as a problem that would affect your well-being in surgery, she talks to the anesthesiologist and the surgeon. They discuss treatment options, additional tests, and whether the surgery should be postponed or canceled. If treatment is started for a specific problem, you will be rechecked to see if it's having the desired effect and then you are cleared for surgery.

Anesthesia Evaluation

When you come in for pre-surgical testing, you also meet with an anesthesiologist or other representative from the anesthesiology department. This is your opportunity to ask questions of the specialist who administers anesthesia, though not necessarily from the same doctor who will be present at your operation.

Every patient should be given the option to have this meeting in advance of the day of surgery. Unfortunately, this doesn't always happen. Your surgeon is the one to refer you, but not all of them do it. The anesthesiologist isn't going to seek you out the week before surgery and say, "Hey, I haven't met you yet. Come in and let's talk about how we can numb you up." *You* have to take the initiative and say, "I want to discuss my surgery with a member of the anesthesia department before the day of my operation." When you schedule your pre-surgical tests, be sure to schedule a visit with the anesthesiologist.

If you don't talk to an anesthesiologist in advance, the first time you will meet her is within minutes of your surgery. This is not ideal from anyone's perspective. Sure, anesthesiologists are highly trained professionals who know what to do from reading your chart, medical history, and vital signs. And you are still awake and can ask questions. But what other critically important matter do you leave until immediately before the point of no return? If you're buying a house, would you wait until ten minutes before closing to talk to the building inspector?

An advance meeting gives everyone a chance to evaluate the situation. The anesthesiologist or staff member will want to find out your past medical history, previous surgery, what kind of anesthesia you've had, how you reacted to it, your current medical condition, what medication you are taking. And you want to know what kinds of anesthesia are available and what their pros and cons are. You can ask questions like: will I feel anything, remember the surgery, wake up unexpectedly, or have side effects? Also, make sure that any doctor who will administer and monitor your anesthesia is board-certified in anesthesiology.

It's comforting to know this in advance of your surgery. When the day comes, the anesthesiologist reviews your condition and relevant additional information; you raise any questions you still have. If you've met previously, there's much less likelihood of surprises for either of you on the day of surgery.

For example, a patient who had undergone multiple surgeries on his back was planning to have an operation for a condition unrelated to his back problems and for which the usual anesthetic was a spinal. However, because of those previous surgeries, at the presurgical visit the anesthesiologist determined that a spinal was not the best choice. She recommended general anesthesia instead. The patient had time to talk about what the differences between the two types were and why general anesthesia was better for him. When he arrived the day of surgery, the patient was mentally prepared to receive general anesthesia.

Don't let fears about anesthesia plague you in the days or weeks before surgery. Deal with your imagined terrors by getting as full an understanding of the scientific realities as you feel you need. Chapter 10 describes the different types of anesthesia in detail and why they are used.

THE NIGHT BEFORE SURGERY

It is very rare today to be admitted for any type of surgery the night before unless there is a compelling reason. For example, a patient with heart problems was at risk because she was taken off her usual medication in preparation for surgery. The cardiologist said she had to be closely monitored and her insurance plan agreed to cover the charges from the hospital for the earlier admission.

But a phone call from the hospital the night before is customary. You will be told by a member of the hospital staff what time to arrive, what you need to pay, if anything, and your doctor's orders, including no eating or drinking twelve hours prior to surgery. In this call, it is likely you will hear things that you've heard at least a few times before in the doctor's office, in written material, and at presurgical testing. No one on the surgeon's staff or in the hospital wants to leave to guesswork questions like: "Do you think the patient will show up for surgery?" or "Wonder if she forgot to fast and had bacon and eggs for breakfast?"

CHECKING IN
Arrival

Usually you arrive at the hospital about one to three hours before you have surgery. You are instructed to go to a designated registration area, identify yourself, and provide your insurance information. You will be given information and booklets about your hospital stay. Then you will be escorted either to the ambulatory surgery area if you are going home the same day or to the OR suite if you're staying over.

For day surgery, you'll be brought to a room that is like a holding area, where you take off your street clothes and put on a hospital gown and an identification bracelet. You will be asked questions by the staff, such as, "When did you last eat or take medications?" and "How are you feeling?" The anesthesiologist will speak to you again to make sure nothing has changed. You can have the support of a friend or family member throughout this part of the surgical process. You should not be told you have to wait alone, and if a doctor wants privacy to examine you, for example, your companion can step outside. Usually only one person is allowed in; once you are ready to enter the operating room, your friend or family member will be sent to a waiting room.

Payment and Insurance

When you check in, your insurance information is verified. This data has already been passed along by your doctor's office and is in the hospital computer. You will confirm that nothing has changed, or if it has, supply the new information.

If your insurance coverage requires a deductible or copayment, you pay it at this time, by cash, check, or credit card. This shouldn't be a surprise. As an informed consumer, know the details of your plan and what you are required to pay. When the hospital receives approval of your surgery from the insurance company, the payment and reimbursement arrangements are reviewed and you will be reminded of them in the phone call you receive from the hospital the night before surgery.

In the course of your hospital stay, you will incur charges from different departments. You may not understand why bills are being mailed directly to you from the radiology or pathology departments. Even though the hospital has your insurance information, it does not necessarily get to every billing entity in the hospital. You know you're covered, but the bills keep coming. Simply photocopy your insurance card and send it back together with the bill to clear the matter up—or call their billing office with the information.

Since you have surgery on the same day as you arrive, you don't want to hassle over insurance coverage then. Make it your business to have the details taken care of in advance so that the only thing left on the day of your surgery is simple verification of the accuracy of the data. It can be very upsetting to deal with bureaucracies or feel you are being treated unfairly. This is not where your attention should be at this point.

Consent Forms

If you have been an active consumer in the process from the beginning, signing the consent forms is a pro forma act, not a revelation. Doctors get your verbal consent in advance; some also have you sign the consent form in their office, and then sign it again at the hospital on the day of surgery. Be well prepared for this moment. This is the acknowledgment that you do know the alternatives and the risks and benefits of the operation, and that you're having it willingly.

Consent forms may be difficult to read or lack detail, but states generally require certain basic information, and an expiration date. At this time there is no simplified form that is in general use. Even though you've discussed your surgery, if there's still something in the form you don't understand, ask for an explanation before you sign it. (A sample consent form can be found in Appendix D on pages 325–26.)

Personal Items: What to Bring

You need documents related to your surgery, primarily your insurance card and your instructions. If you have a health-care proxy form or a living will, hand those over at admitting. (See Chapter 5 for more discussion on these matters.) Keep copies of them with you or give them to a relative or friend. It's helpful to have a credit card to pay for TV service or other small items (if your stay will be overnight), but try to have a family member take care of that so you don't have to be concerned about hanging on to your credit card.

The only clothes you really need are a bathrobe, slippers, and underwear. As soon as you're well enough to wear street clothes, you're probably already on your way home. You can either keep a set of clothes in the closet of your hospital room or arrange to have someone bring them when you're ready to leave. Although there's nothing fashionable about hospital gowns, they have proven over time to be the most practical solution to the question of how to cover your body while it is hooked up to tubes and you're dealing with drains and dressings. You couldn't get in and out of most regular clothing, nor do you want blood or other fluids staining them. While you may bemoan the time you wear the hospital johnny, you'll also find it's the most comfortable alternative.

It's a good idea to bring your favorite soap and toothpaste. Toiletries are available at the hospital and they will be brought to you if you need them. But why wait for them, pay for them, or get ones you don't like when you can easily pack a few of these essential items?

Bring personal belongings that give you positive reinforcement, like reading material, music, a photo, an item of spiritual support like a rosary or a focal point for meditation. But don't bring something of great value. As in any place where many people come and go, your object of value left unattended can become someone else's object of temptation. You may be out of your room for periods at a time, or you may have to switch rooms. Costly electronic equipment, for example, may break, get lost, or disappear. You could be on painkillers and fall asleep, so your disc player slips off the bed and onto the floor. Leave your treasures at home. You will probably have visitors, so if you have neglected to take something that brings you comfort, someone can bring it to you after your surgery.

NEXT STEPS

These preparations are designed to make your surgery as successful as possible. It may seem like a lot to leave no stone unturned, but each ingredient—deciding to have surgery, finding the right surgeon, and arranging for tests, insurance, and the details of your hospital stay—contributes to a great outcome.

In Part Three, surgeons from several specialties at Columbia Presbyterian Center provided information to describe in plain English what you need to know if you, or someone close to you, is going to have any one of the forty-five most common operations. In the following chapters, I will describe what to expect in recovery and what to plan for during discharge and your return home. If you are trying to learn a good golf swing you've heard it's all in the follow-through. Similarly, in surgery it is not only what happens in preparation, or even in the actual operation that counts. The aftermath is also essential to your healing. Dealing with recovery and pain and working out the best discharge plan are important parts of the surgical process as a whole.

8

What to Expect in Recovery

Often, the aftermath of surgery is little more than an afterthought. But unless you focus on it early on, you're vulnerable to learning later that once the operation ends, another ordeal can begin.

Doctors also may downplay the effects that even routine surgery has on the body. The same surgeon who gives you a detailed description of the diagnosis and operation may dismiss recovery with a few cursory remarks. That sounds reasonable when you're sitting in his office clothed and fairly comfortable, but it's not helpful when you come out of an operation and wonder what's next.

When one patient decided to have surgery for her hemorrhoids, she figured it would be just like the procedure she had in her doctor's office several years earlier. She'd get the problem fixed and then for a short time after, feel a little uncomfortable from the effects of the treatment.

A professional woman who routinely does research as part of her job, she said her surgeon's office glossed over the recovery by telling her that she'd be uncomfortable the first week, much better the second, and fine by the third. That piece of information, and a yellowed photocopy of an instruction sheet with her medication schedule penciled in, was all the detail she had about what to expect after surgery.

But her recovery didn't turn out as she had expected. For weeks, even months, after the outpatient surgery in a nearby hospital, she felt exhausted. She went home after the surgery nauseated and vomiting. She wasn't warned about the discharge she was having from the wound, nor was she given anything helpful like a pad to wear for her trip home from the hospital. While those were temporary problems, she experienced intense long-term cramping from intestinal gas and the need to go to the bathroom instantly when the first urges struck. Instead of heading back to work within twenty-four hours, as the instruction sheet said, she could do little more than remain housebound on a reclining chair.

Before the operation she didn't press her doctor about recovery or do independent research. As she'd had the same procedure before, she logically assumed it would be the same, and she'd have an easy time. It was a surprise when, after the operation, she had problems with gas and elimination, an inability to return to her usual routines, and a big question: "Why?"

INFORMATION

Surgery is an ever-evolving field of medicine, and things may have changed dramatically since you last had an operation, or heard the tales of someone else who did. For example, today you can administer your own pain medication intravenously, whenever you feel you need it, through a calibrated pump at your bedside; you can eliminate the trouble of caring for dressings since most wounds now don't require them; and you can have an easier time with personal care since you typically shower within forty-eight hours instead of waiting weeks.

If you sense an information gap, you can take the initiative and find out details like what usually happens in recovery and what is unlikely, but possible. It's not out of place to ask. The recovery process is different for each patient in each operation. It is better to dig a little than end up being uninformed about the post-surgical experience.

A heart surgeon was operated on to repair his shoulder. He knew all about the aftermath of a coronary bypass—but not the aftermath of shoulder surgery. He was prepared for pain, but not for the fact that his rehabilitation meant six full months of physical therapy.

What could he—and you—do differently? Ask the experts. If your surgeon tells you that you'll have to have physical therapy after the operation, get clear, thorough answers to questions like: "Will I have to travel to a medical facility or do the exercises at home? How many times a week? How many weeks? Will I have pain while doing the exercises? What kind of progress should I expect to make in my range of motion? When can I go back to my job full-time? Will I be able to play my favorite sport? Lift groceries? When can I expect to be 'normal' as I define it in my lifestyle?"

Your surgeon may not even have enough information. Take his remarks as a compass, pointing you to the source for more. Tell him you understand you'll need physical therapy. Can he give you the name and number of the person in the hospital's physical-therapy department who treats patients recovering from your particular type of surgery?

Instead of feeling more anxiety, patients often say they are more confident when they find out the whole picture, especially since they are also learning techniques that help them feel better.

Once again, you're a consumer involved in making a major purchase for your health. If you were buying a car, wouldn't you want to know how it would run before you left the showroom? You'd find out whether you're likely to get ten or twenty-two miles to the gallon of gas. Similarly, after your operation you want to know whether you'll be confined to a chair for days or dancing the polka next week, and why.

PHYSICAL EFFECTS

The most long-lasting effect of surgery is often fatigue. It varies in intensity by the medical condition of the patient and type of operation, but it's common in all types of operations. The symptoms that you experience sound vague—you don't feel well and you tire easily—but they are very real. Although the medical problem that caused you to have surgery has been corrected, you don't feel up to snuff—at least not yet.

An operation, even a minor one, inflicts trauma that often leaves you debilitated, depleted, and disoriented. Your body has passed through a series of hits: you've been cut, starved, and knocked out by powerful drugs. The sedation and painkillers given with local anesthesia are often strong enough to put your body out of action for a time. If you had general anesthesia the reaction is more intense. During surgery, your chest muscles and diaphragm weren't bringing air in and out of your body; a breathing machine was doing that work for you. In fact your whole system was shut down, and the full functioning of muscles like those in your stomach and intestines take time to come back. Think about how you sometimes feel after just one cocktail. Narcotics like morphine are only one of the drugs you're taking during a short period of time. Its effects are much more potent than one cocktail.

And you expected to get up right again and act as usual, marked only by a bandage and a Tylenol? Anyone who's gone through surgery knows the piece-of-cake recovery is often up there with Santa Claus and the Easter bunny in the realm of myths. If you think you won't have any major discomfort just because no one told you about it, remember that not every medical professional is forthcoming about the details.

Research has shown that, post-operatively, the mental and physical abilities of many people are so affected by surgery that they cannot return easily or quickly to their normal routines. Reaction times and ability to coordinate motor skills are still often out of whack for weeks. What does that mean? Things you do automatically, like driving a car, may be more of a strain for a while.

In one study, people who had surgery were observed for their reaction times. Among other tests, they were given a sheet of nonsense letters, scrambled in groups of three. They were told to pick out as many letters on the sheet that were arranged in a certain order, like the letters "adr," within thirty seconds.

The study showed it was hardest to do this task four or five days after surgery. However, some patients continued to have difficulty three, even six weeks after surgery. So don't be surprised if you come out of surgery feeling slower and less efficient. It should not be permanent.

EMOTIONAL EFFECTS

You—and your family—may also wonder why, after surgery, you're getting so angry at little things. After all, the surgery was a success. Why are you being so difficult? Understand that mood swings are one of the byproducts of surgery. A classic experiment done in the 1960s helps to explain why.

College students were asked to participate in a study that looked at the effect of a certain vitamin on vision. Instead of a vitamin, the unsuspecting participants were given an injection of a small dose of epinephrine, which is adrenaline. Others got a saline injection, given as a control since it had no effects on the students. (Under today's more stringent rules, misleading the subjects about what they were taking wouldn't pass muster. The results of the experiment, however, are worth noting.)

The students were then observed as they sat in a waiting room. Seated next to each student was a person who was planted there to act either as a happy, animated companion, or as a depressed person. The experiment showed those students who got adrenaline and were interacting with a happy person became *extremely* happy. If a student was seated next to someone who was depressed, then he became very down, too. Compared to those on adrenaline, the students who got saline solutions had much less of a reaction to either type of person.

During the surgical process your natural levels of adrenaline go up, a reaction that's often referred to as the stress response. Adrenaline is just one of the powerful chemicals that flow through your body during sedation, anesthesia, and pain control. Any one of those drugs may be having an effect on your emotional state, causing wider mood swings.

There's plenty of opportunity to play out those emotions. You're in a confined and unfamiliar room, visited by anxious relatives. You have to interact with strangers on the staff for your basic needs. It all can be enormously comforting, or totally infuriating. Many patients, their families, and even their doctors do not grasp what that can feel like.

The best way to prepare is to recognize that these reactions are common after surgery. Remind yourself that the operation is a ticket to health, not sainthood.

There are ways to feel better that do not involve adding more drugs to the mix. Staying calm through complementary-medicine techniques, prayer, caring companions, and positive thinking can help you emerge from surgery feeling more in control and up to the challenges. These will be discussed further in Chapter 9. For now, let's look more at recovery, intensive care, and pain control.

THE RECOVERY ROOM

"Can you hear me? How do you feel?" The surgeon may use the most high-tech equipment available for your surgery, but when it comes to making sure you're conscious, the most common tool is the human voice.

Expect to wake up in the OR to a hello from someone on the operating team. At that point, general anesthesia has stopped and the breathing tube, if you had one, has been generally removed. If you had a local anesthetic in addition to sedation, you're also prodded awake and spoken to in the OR. You'll be groggy and you probably won't remember waking up because the medications you've had induce amnesia.

Once it's been determined that you can respond, you'll be taken to the recovery room. Under certain circumstances, some patients go to the intensive-care unit, a more detailed monitoring area, which I'll discuss later.

Patients are monitored for vital signs and bleeding in the recovery room. In a large hospital, there may be several recovery rooms, each with space for about fifteen patients. At Columbia-Presbyterian, each room is monitored by a recovery-room team of anesthesiologists, attending doctors, residents, and nurses.

Patients are hooked up to monitors, including an EKG to monitor heart rate and rhythm and a monitor on a finger to measure oxygen. The nurse takes the patient's blood pressure, initially every 5 minutes, increasing to every 15 minutes or so. There is typically one nurse to about every two or three patients.

Recovery-room procedures pick up where the operating room left off, with pain medication. Usually at this point a narcotic like morphine is given intravenously and you'll be drowsy, but conscious.

If you are an outpatient, that is, an ambulatory patient who is going to leave the hospital on the same day as your surgery, you have to meet certain criteria before being allowed to leave. You need to be able to walk and urinate on your own, and your pain should be manageable. If you are staying in the hospital, you are not released to the regular floor until your vital signs are stable, pain is under control, and you are aware enough that someone doesn't have to constantly tap you awake. Depending on the nature of the surgery and anesthesia, this could take anywhere from 30 minutes to 6 or 7 hours.

The surgeon may stop in to check on you, and then go to see your family in the waiting area to update them on the operation. Generally, the family can visit the patient in the recovery room, even if it's in the middle of the night. They may be allowed to stay for brief intervals, or longer, depending on the hospital's policies. Check in advance with your surgeon to find out how long visitors can stay in the recovery room.

If recovery progresses smoothly, vital signs are good, the anesthesiologist clears you, and a bed is available on the regular floor, you are transferred to your room on a stretcher by an attendant. This should not be a difficult experience. A nurse on the floor should be expecting your arrival and be able to attend to you as soon as you arrive. Generally, you do not see a doctor at this point.

After you go to your hospital room, you should continue to be watched closely. The doctor will write instructions to the staff telling them to check vital signs at certain intervals. This is a time when the general quality of care in an institution shows its face. Budget cuts have hit the nursing staffs of hospitals hard and one result is that the ratio of patients to nurses has gone up; ten or twelve patients to one nurse is not unusual on a hospital floor.

The highest ranking nurse is the RN (registered nurse). In descending order of skills and training, there are LPNs (licensed practical nurses), nurses aides, and patient-care associates. This last group is trained to perform basic techniques in an abbreviated course that may run a couple of months. They don't have the depth of medical training of either an RN or LPN. You may not know whether you are being cared for by an RN or an associate. Ideally, the person should introduce himself, but this doesn't always happen. If you have any question about what a person is doing, ask who he is and why he is doing it.

This is the time during which some patients arrange for a private-duty nurse, at their own expense. Others have family members available to keep a close watch. The amount of time a family member is present may be limited by hospital policies; for example, if another patient is in the room, the family may not be allowed to stay if it's past visiting hours. On the other hand, sometimes relatives are permitted practically to move in with you.

It is likely that you will be expected to get up the next day and start moving, even if it's uncomfortable for you. There is an urgency to this so you don't develop problems with your lungs, or with blood clots in the veins of your legs. You'll be asked to cough, do deep breathing, expand your lungs and get up, with help if necessary, to sit in a chair or take a few steps. You may be given stockings to wear that inflate and decompress gently to help prevent blood clots. You may be turned in bed if you can't do it on your own, after a hip replacement, for example, so that you don't get bedsores.

In the hours and days after surgery, you may experience the effects of the surgery itself, feel nauseated from anesthesia, and have a sore throat from the breathing tube. You may also be constipated from the pain medication. It takes time after the anesthesia for the muscles to get up to speed, so your stomach and intestines may not be functioning normally yet and you won't be able to eat. The nurse will check for gurgling sounds in your stomach to see if the juices are flowing again. Patients usually start out with clear fluids: first ice chips, a little bit of water, then apple juice, tea, or broth. If you can hold those down, then you progress to cereal or other simple, soft foods.

INTENSIVE-CARE UNIT (ICU)

The main reason you'd go to an intensive-care unit after surgery is that you are at risk for serious, and generally treatable, medical problems after surgery.

Certain surgeries, like a cardiac bypass or major vascular surgery, automatically require patients to recover in an ICU. Other patients are sent there because even though their surgery doesn't call for it, the general state of their health is precarious enough to require constant monitoring. In both of these circumstances, you know in advance that you'll be going to the ICU.

Sometimes, however, the trip to the ICU is unforeseen. The decision to send a patient to the ICU is made by the anesthesiologist and the surgeon. There may have been a complication during surgery, due to the patient's other health problems, the operation, or the anesthesia. For instance, a patient undergoing a hysterectomy could have unexpected bleeding during the operation and would need to be monitored carefully afterward.

The difference between intensive care and a regular recovery room is the number of medical personnel available and the intensity of the monitoring. For example, in a regular recovery room, the blood pressure is monitored at intervals by means of a blood-pressure cuff, the familiar technique from doctor's visits; in an ICU, a catheter is placed in the artery in the wrist and blood pressure is monitored continuously. Every heartbeat is projected on a screen with a blood-pressure reading. Catheters may also go into the heart and monitor the heart pressure, after bypass surgery for example, Patients may remain on a breathing machine, at least for a few hours after surgery. Besides the basic monitoring of blood pressure, pulse, breathing, temperature, and oxygen level, there may be additional observation that is specific to a patient's case, such as testing for neurological functioning.

The design of an ICU and the number of beds varies by hospital. Some hospitals have different ICUs for different types of surgeries. An ICU may be as small as four beds, or as large as thirty. In most of them, the patients occupy private cubicles or rooms, separated from other patients by some form of partition.

When a patient first arrives in the ICU, it usually takes about half an hour for the team to hook him up to the monitors, draw blood, and get him stabilized. As long as the patient doesn't need emergency care such as resuscitation techniques, the family can come into the ICU to visit.

The idea of being sent to the ICU may seem alarming, especially if it's due to a complication, but you are assured of special monitoring and care. While they are there, patients may be aware of their surroundings, but initially they are often heavily sedated to tolerate the breathing tube that may remain in place. It's uncomfortable, since the tube goes through your mouth and down your windpipe. But because the sedation causes some amnesia, you may not remember it was there.

Patients are usually in the ICU for a day or two; some patients remain for weeks or months, but that is not common.

There's a lot of state-of-the-art equipment in intensive care. When you are well enough, or if your family is interested, find out from the staff why certain things are hooked up to you and what they do. For example, the patch on your chest monitors your heart rhythm and the tape on your finger is a pulse oximeter that measures the degree to which your red blood cells are saturated with oxygen. Which waves and numbers on the screen are your blood pressure, your heart rate? You and your family can tune in to what the numbers mean as you progress through intensive care.

At some point, often a day or two after surgery, you will be considered well enough to go to a regular hospital room and continue your recovery there.

PAIN

One of the biggest fears for a patient making the journey from the operating room to his own living room is pain. Rest assured that virtually all pain can be now controlled with a large array of drugs. There is no reason for you to be in agony after an operation.

Still, studies continue to show that after surgery patients are undermedicated for pain. Don't let that happen to you. If you think either that you're supposed to bite the bullet and be in pain, or that enduring pain is better than taking any more narcotics, strike both of those thoughts. Being a stoic is not helpful; in fact, it can be the reverse. If you have so much pain that you can't take a deep breath or cough, then you're hurting yourself. You have to cough after surgery so that your lungs are kept clear and you don't end up with pneumonia or a collapsed lung. If pain prevents you from coughing, you need relief so you can clear your lungs.

So little attention has been paid to the question of pain relief after surgery that the federal government's Agency for Health Care Policy Research (AHCPR) has taken up the issue. The agency, which studies high-frequency problems that could benefit from a policy statement, has emphasized a more aggressive approach to pain after surgery, through more frequent assessment of a patient's level of pain by health-care professionals, more patient involvement in pain control.

Just as you have throughout the process of surgery, take on the issue of pain management as your own. Make sure you understand that you should not be in pain, it can be harmful to your recovery, and there are plenty of pharmacological options available to remove the pain. Learn how pain is generally managed for your type of surgery. Find out who can adjust your medication if it is inadequate. And feel confident that being proactive about pain management is a step in the right direction.

Pain control actually starts in the operating room. In some cases, pain medications are administered during surgery and carry through into the recovery room, ICU, or hospital floor. For example, in prostate surgery, an epidural catheter may be inserted into a space in the patient's back. This catheter supplies medication during surgery and as the area is already numbed and the catheter in place, the introduction of pain medication during surgery is done easily. Since the medication starts before the patient wakes up and is supplied continuously through the catheter, at no point does the patient have to experience pain. This method is particularly helpful during the worst of the pain, which often lasts through the first two days after surgery.

Similarly, if you have arm surgery with regional anesthesia, when the anesthetic is injected in the shoulder, a long-lasting pain medication can be injected as well. This will last for the twenty-four hours when the pain is the worst; by the time it wears off, you are likely to be over the most painful period, and less potent oral medications are enough.

The amount and duration of pain medication varies for each patient and each type of operation. In a cataract operation, for example, the level of associated pain is usually fairly low, almost nonexistent. Surgery on bones, on the other hand, can be quite painful for days, even weeks. Get an idea how much pain is associated with your surgery, and qualify that information by recognizing that pain control is an individual issue. Don't suffer in silence and don't try to be heroic about pain.

If something hurts, state that directly and clearly: "I have pain." If what you've been given isn't working, then say you want to try something else. Hospitals like Columbia-Presbyterian have experts in pain management, who go in teams to evaluate a patient's pain situation and prescribe the medication to alleviate it. They are available around the clock to see patients, look for side effects, and adjust medications.

Pain usually begins in the very early period after an operation, but may be worse a day or two later due to swelling and inflammation. The first pain medication you receive may be the narcotic morphine, or the synthetic narcotic Demerol; these are administered intravenously. After the most intense pain diminishes, you can generally manage it with less powerful oral medications. These include acetaminophen, whose brand names include Tylenol. It is often used in combination with codeine. There are also ibuprofen drugs like Motrin and Advil; older anti-inflammatory drugs like aspirin; and a newer class of anti-inflammatory drugs like Toradol, which can be quite strong.

One of the most reassuring and common ways of dealing with pain is to control the medication yourself. A device, called a PCA pump, which stands for patient-controlled analgesia, lets you get pain medication as soon as you need it. At the push of a button, you can self-administer a measured dose of morphine or Demerol, which is then delivered intravenously. There are built-in safeguards so you don't overdose. The dosage is premeasured and you can only access it at a specified interval of, say, every six minutes. The device is easy to operate, even for someone coming out of surgery. Since all you have to do is hit a button, you can start using it in the recovery room right after you wake up.

Perhaps you've had an orthopedic operation with local anesthesia and now the numbness is wearing off and you are beginning to feel pain. You're in the recovery room, the PCA pump is next to you, and set up for your use. You hit the button when you feel you need it and a measured dose of morphine is delivered to you immediately. The next time you need the medicine again is up to you; it could be thirty minutes, or three hours, depending on your individual pain threshold. You don't have to call a doctor or nurse . . . then wait.

Studies are showing that patients actually end up using less medicine when they administer it themselves. When timing is not an issue—you get medication as soon as you need it—then the dosage you need is not as high. Also, there is a feeling of security when you know you are in charge of relieving your own pain.

For any drug that is potent as a painkiller, there are side effects. The most dangerous is that excessive pain medication can kill you. If you take an overdose of narcotics, you stop breathing. But in a hospital setting, you are monitored and there is a built-in margin of safety in the amounts that you are given.

Other side effects include impaired functioning, delirium, constipation, and nausea. Pain medications are often given in combination with other drugs to block those reactions. Constipation is probably the most common. Lying in bed, not drinking water, and taking pain medications is a recipe for constipation. Although it's not generally something you fear after surgery, it can be a bigger problem, and make you more uncomfortable than pain.

One generally overblown fear is that as a result of taking narcotic painkillers after an operation, you will become addicted to them. Under normal circumstances you can use these drugs on a short-term basis and not develop a physiological craving for them.

There are exceptions, however. If you have a history of alcoholism or drug abuse, for example, then you and your doctor are at a different level of decision making about whether you can become addicted to pain medication.

First of all, recognize that even with such a history, you should not deny yourself strong pain medication in the early period after an operation. But the transition to less intense pain medicines that are not addicting—drugs like Tylenol, aspirin, ibuprofen—should be as early as possible. If you do go home still taking a drug like Percocet, which contains a synthetic narcotic, you would not get a refill without first consulting with your doctor. Refills are unusual and are, of course, controlled by the physician. Repeated requests for refills for a drug that has the potential to be addicting would draw a response from any good physician.

Whatever your concern, don't build up a phobia. Instead find out what medication and resources are available. Some problems, pain included, can be helped by a combination of drugs and other techniques like relaxation.

Some people can distance themselves from pain without medication. An extreme example is in China, where major surgery is done on patients who are awake, with their pain controlled through acupuncture. Whether internally generated substances like endorphins, which are responsible for the "runner's high," could be turned on by people to reduce pain is a topic that is still largely unknown.

Massage can also help in pain control because it reduces soreness and helps you relax. Other approaches that some find valuable for reducing pain include yoga, deep breathing, and hypnotherapy. If you want to learn more about different ways to relax, consult with practitioners of these techniques, ideally before the operation. Tell your surgeon about any alternative methods of pain control you're using.

Don't get down on yourself if you haven't been able to use anything but medication. It is misguided to think that control of strong pain without drugs is an option for most patients; the question of what else works has not yet been verified.

It's normal that questions about recovery and pain control after surgery may not yet be uppermost in your mind, since you've focused on the disease and the operation. It's similar to a woman who's going to have a baby. There's a lot of attention on the birth and delivery before it happens. But once the baby is born and before you can even catch your breath, the delivery passes into history and then you have to go home and raise the kid. Likewise, once your operation is over, you've got to take the effects of the surgery home with you and learn to deal with them. By taking the time now, and in the hospital after surgery, you can eliminate surprises and put the healing process more firmly into your hands.

Your attitude, efforts to plan a quality discharge program, and commitment to caring for yourself all combine with your surgeon's best efforts to make your surgical process a success.

9

Coping in the Aftermath
of Surgery

If you start discharge planning early you can depart with a minimum of stress. It's not possible to know in advance of an operation everything that will happen after it, but you certainly can have a realistic understanding of your own circumstances and the typical needs of a patient who's had an operation like yours.

Most patients fall into one of the following categories:

1. *People who leave the hospital under their own steam.* This group can include those who've had simple surgery to patients who've had more complex operations such as heart surgery. Usually, though, these are younger and healthier patients who've had routine surgery, like removal of a cyst. They need some help from family or friends, especially to drive them home, stay with them until they're comfortable, and supply food and medical items. Although these patients, too, feel effects like fatigue, their discharge planning is at a minimum.

2. *People who have more complex medical and social problems.* They go home but need more skilled assistance, a visiting nurse, for example, who comes to check on an incision. They may need special equipment, like a wheelchair. Discharge planning is necessary to make arrangements with an agency to provide

nursing and physical therapy-visits and for ordering equipment and instructing patients on its use. Such patients need a companion to stay with them and may have to be transported home in an ambulette (a vehicle that accommodates patients who can sit up, such as those in a wheelchair, but who can't maneuver into a car). An ambulance is necessary when a person has to lie down.

3. *Patients who are ill but can leave the hospital.* Their destination is often a nursing home for long-term care or a rehabilitation facility where they'll have physical, occupational, or speech therapy for a period of time. Consultation with the medical staff is necessary to determine what type of rehab is needed. An acute-care facility provides three to four hours of rehabilitation a day; a subacute about an hour or two daily. This group of patients is often covered by Medicare or Medicaid and the family needs to learn the rules and procedures for coverage under those plans and what facilities are certified to accept patients under federal government guidelines. The social-work department of the hospital will act as an intermediary, finding out information, getting insurance approval, and assuring a bed in the rehabilitation facility.

Before you have your operation, find out the answers to as many questions that are relevant to your discharge. Is it likely that you will go directly home from the hospital, or will you need time in an interim-care facility? How soon after you leave the hospital will you be able to bathe and dress on your own, drive a car, shop for groceries, prepare meals, get to the bank and pharmacy? If you can't do any one of these on your own, who is going to help you? Will family and friends be available, and for how long? Or will you need to hire someone? Does your insurance cover home care and for how many hours or days? Does it pay for equipment like a commode or a walker? When will you be able to resume sexual activity?

Start discussing the matter of your discharge with the social-work department of the medical center before you're even admitted. Your perspective will be clearer, and the social worker's efforts more streamlined. It often takes time to get questions answered through the insurance system. Until now, it's likely you didn't know if your insurance covers a home health aide, for how many visits, and from what agency. You may have a phone number for an insurance-company case manager which, though only a few months old, has already changed about seven times. Your exact post-operative needs may not be known at this early date, but a lot of the grunt work surrounding them can be deftly handled when there is time to do so.

If necessary, social workers can get you out even on a few hours notice. However, if the issues haven't been addressed in advance, you may not get what you want.

Most managed-care companies calculate how long you will stay in the hospital based on guidelines like those published by Milliman & Robertson, an actuarial firm. Such guidelines are increasingly used as benchmarks, but they are not always validated by practical experience. For example, under one set of guidelines, the recommended length of stay for coronary bypass surgery is four days. However, the lowest mortality rates in the country for coronary bypass surgery are in New York State, where the average length of stay is seven to eight days.

Hospital-stay guidelines refer to the average patient. Of course there are always exceptions. Sometimes, the hospital stay is longer than expected because there are complications, like an infection in the wound or a heart ailment that is worsened by the stress of surgery. Sometimes a patient who is doing particularly well may be discharged earlier than planned.

It might be necessary to appeal to the insurance company for additional reimbursement when an individual's case does not fit within an established norm. There are also cases when guidelines have been so flagrantly off the mark that societal protests have been organized to change them. One example is the case of "drive-thru" mastectomies where the guidelines advocated a one-day stay. Now, laws have been enacted to protect the health of patients who have mastectomies by requiring longer stays.

If you have any question about the length of your hospital stay, ask your insurance company to provide you with the source of their decision and any other information on which that decision is based. Discuss the terms with your doctor and find out if she agrees that it is a realistic time frame. Although it surely helps your planning to know in advance just how long you'll be in the hospital, it doesn't help your recovery to leave the hospital before you're medically ready.

Even if discharge is the reasonable next step, you still are tired, your system is not yet operating at normal capacity, and you have to cope with the effects of the operation itself. If you've had eye surgery, you can walk out on your own power, but you can't drive. If you've had knee surgery, you can see fine, but movement is tough. However, if your doctor comes in to your hospital room and says, "Things are looking fine. How'd you like to go home today?" you don't want to hold up your departure because you don't know what's going to happen next. At the very least, you need a companion, transportation, and a place that is safe for you in the aftermath of surgery.

The surgeon decides when you have progressed to the point where the possibility of a serious complication is very low. If you have a fever of 103° F, you will not be sent home; if your wound is still draining and no infection is present, you may be allowed to leave, with instructions on aftercare. Usually the surgeon will tell you when you are ready to be discharged, but the news may also come from another member of the medical team who's been caring for you. Other members of the team, including social workers, nurses, physician's assistants, and residents participate in the decision making and in patient education. Sometimes another doctor, like a specialist in rehabilitation medicine, is called in for a consultation.

ARRANGEMENTS

You bought a surgery package that includes the hospital and staff, and when that staff takes over your discharge planning, you want to be confident that your needs are paramount and their recommendations the best.

Hospital social workers handle hundreds of discharge plans that cover virtually every situation. Personal experience and reference materials provide them with access to resources around the country. And they are trained professionals, often with master's degrees, who can understand your psychological as well as your physical needs.

Hip replacement surgery has repaired your elderly mother's bones after she slipped, fell, and broke her hip. Now that she's well enough to leave the hospital, what happens next? She'd been living on her own until the accident, coping well enough with other chronic health problems like an irregular heartbeat. You're convinced that she can't be alone anymore. But you live a couple of hundred miles away, work full-time, and don't have a clue about what resources are available in her area.

As you try to make arrangements for your mother, whenever you raise the issue of a nursing home, she tells you, "If you loved me, you wouldn't ask me to go there." And when you mention live-in help at home, she says, "I'm not going to let any stranger into my house." You become frustrated, even angry at your mother's stubbornness. You can get the help of a social worker who is skilled in conflict resolution and can talk to your mother about your concern for her safety and your belief that a good nursing home will provide the companionship, activities, and meal preparation she needs. The social worker can go on further to discuss alternatives like adult day-care programs and agencies that provide home health aides after carefully screening them. And she can explore the possibilities of living with a family member, or an assisted-living arrangement.

The social-work department is a major resource for making your transition to the next stage of recovery as easy as possible, from handling the relatively simple appointments for a visiting nurse, to the complex matters of hospice care for the terminally ill and nursing-home placement for the elderly or very sick. If you've stayed overnight for your surgery, you never have to pay extra for social-work services; they are bundled into the rate for the hospital stay. If you are an ambulatory patient who leaves the same day as you have the surgery, and you use a social worker to help arrange your discharge, you may be billed for it. As an outpatient, you usually do not require much assistance from a social worker; however, if you do plan to use their services, check with your insurance to find out if they are covered under your policy.

When a social worker refers you to an agency for nursing care or other services, she is generally using resources that are part of a network approved by the hospital. One of the best ways to judge an agency's performance is through the satisfaction of other customers.

Patients are asked to call the social-work department if something doesn't go right with the services that have been set up for them. Was the nurse in an agency usually late, rude, or too hasty in her care? Patient feedback helps the hospital staff to know whether to recommend an agency again.

Of course, mistakes happen. One of the criteria that experienced social workers will use in evaluating an agency is whether, when something does go wrong, the staff recognizes it and fixes it. When one patient needed a piece of equipment delivered to her home so she could be discharged, her family became more frantic as the time for discharge neared and the equipment hadn't arrived yet. Since the nursing agency chosen to provide the skilled services at home was responsible for ordering the equipment, they got right on the case. The agency staff called the vendor who replied that they hadn't delivered the equipment because they hadn't received payment yet from the patient's HMO. The nursing agency, in turn, guaranteed payment and insisted that the equipment be delivered immediately.

The agency didn't drop the matter at that point. They sent a letter to the hospital explaining what happened and a complaint to the vendor with notification that in the future, the vendor had to notify the agency in a timely manner about any payment problems. Although a patient or her family can't know the history and response patterns of agencies, a good hospital social-work department keeps on top of this and knows who to recommend from past experience.

Of course, many patients fall under the constraints of medical insurance requirements. Sometimes a managed-care company will only do business with certain agencies. What if you are going to be discharged tomorrow, you need a nurse's visit, and your managed-care company will only reimburse nurses from XYZ agency? The social worker at the hospital calls XYZ and they say it's impossible to send a nurse tomorrow. So the social worker calls your insurance company back and says how about sending ABC agency instead? Some companies will agree; others won't. Instead of sending you home with no one to help you, the social worker can try to make adjustments, like delaying the hour of your discharge so the hospital nurse can change your dressing just before you leave.

Sometimes a patient goes home but is terminally ill. There are hospice programs that can help such patients stay at home as long as possible with the help of specially trained nurses, religious counselors, and social workers. For one mother in her forties, a recurrence of cancer that spread from her breast to her brain meant she wouldn't live much longer. At first, she went home with the help of hospice care. As she became weaker, it was too hard on her and her teenage children for her to remain there.

The social-work staff at the hospital where she first had her surgery knew of a nearby hospital that cared only for terminally ill cancer patients and that had special pain-management programs for them. During the last six weeks of her life, the patient chose to live there. Her children were able to visit her in an atmosphere that provided the kind of comfort and support they needed and that helped diffuse the frustration of no longer being able to help her at home.

Most people don't know about specialized resources such as a hospital for cancer patients in the last stages of life. You can do independent research, but you don't need to reinvent the wheel when it comes to finding resources in the community for your particular situation. Social workers are there to help fulfill your needs in the aftermath of surgery.

NEXT

Before you leave the hospital, you sign a discharge form; one copy goes home with you and another stays in your chart. Be very clear about what you are allowed to do and what could be harmful: complete instructions for caring for the area that was operated on; the warning signs like bleeding, fever, temperature, or additional pain that tell you it's time to call the surgeon; the best time to have the first routine visit with the surgeon.

Nurses have traditionally been the major resource for providing detailed information on aftercare. But nursing staffs have been cut back at many hospitals. When it comes to responding to a patient in difficulty and one who needs to review an instruction sheet, a short-handed staff has little choice but to get to the emergencies first.

Once again, be persistent and ask questions until you get answers, to lifestyle as well as medical questions. When can you go back to work, resume sex, exercise, travel? If you had surgery for cancer and just learned you have to have chemotherapy because the cancer has spread, it can be very hard to pay full attention to topics like when you can shower. But you need to know the details for when you're back at home. Your family can help by listening to the instructions and by tracking down the medical personnel who have answers. Visiting hours aren't only a time for banter. You might be confined to the bed but your sister can step down to the nurses' station and buttonhole the nurse on your behalf.

The following are a few of the issues you want cleared up before you leave the hospital.

Caring for Your Surgical Incision

A nurse or other qualified professional should teach you this. Even if you will have some skilled care at home, you should know what's going on. For example, if the surgeon leaves the wound open a little and packs it in with gauze and sterile water, the gauze may be changed by a visiting nurse. However, you need to know signs of trouble. If your insurance will not cover nursing visits, you may have to learn the process yourself. If you are squeamish or otherwise unable to do it, you have to either get a family member or friend to help you, or you may have to pay privately for a health aide.

In some cases, such as a stomach tumor removal or lymph-node removal for breast cancer, the patient goes home with a drainage apparatus. The surgeon and the nurses explain what any tubes are for, what color the liquid that will drain into the tube should be, how to measure the output, and how to change the dressing. They'll also review showering and how to keep the hands clean and the area sterile.

After other surgeries, including many heart operations, patients no longer wear dressings. By the time they go home, the wound is closed surgically and it is dry. In the past, patients were told not to take a shower after heart surgery for at least six weeks. That's changed dramatically. Now many surgeons believe you don't need to stew in your own juices and that it is safe to shower or bathe within forty-eight hours after the operation. Speak to your surgeon to find out what her instructions are and why.

Nutrition

You may feel, with good reason, that you need to pay close attention to what you eat in the aftermath of surgery. What food can you tolerate, and what builds up your strength? Even if there are no dietary rules in connection with your type of surgery, you may want to do more than just go back to your regular eating patterns.

Some doctors put nutrition high on their list of priorities for their patients and help them explore how vitamins, nutritional supplements, and food can help them heal. If this appeals to you, find a doctor or other informed source you feel you can trust to get this information. Other doctors caution that scientific research to justify adhering to any particular regimen of supplements is poor or nonexistent.

Exercise

What kind of movements or lifting you can do after surgery, from whether you can walk unaided to how soon you'll be back to the barbells, varies. Talk openly with your surgeon about what is reasonable and what isn't, and why. If you need physical therapy, leave the hospital with a referral for starting your prescribed regimen of recovery exercises.

Work and Play

Some people have a hernia operation on Friday and are back to work on Monday. For others, the discomfort persists weeks later. In other surgeries, like removing part of the liver, recovery will take months while the liver regenerates. How soon and how completely you resume your lifestyle depends on the kind of surgery you're having and the general state of your physical and psychological health. Let your surgeon and her staff know what your concerns are and find out the professional response given your surgery and physical capabilities.

YOUR ROLE

Even if it's been tough for you to go through the surgical experience, you've probably felt some benefit from being in the cocoonlike setting of a hospital. Your medical needs have top priority there; now you must reenter the mainstream where the story of your surgery has to contend with the rest of life for attention. Furthermore, the operation was successful in fixing your problem, but you don't feel like yourself yet.

You may not even be able to go directly home since you have to have rehab, requiring you adjust to a new facility all over again. The need for this alternative varies widely by type of surgery, age, and support systems. If you've fractured your pelvis, it's difficult to go directly home from the hospital. If you're twenty-one and live at home, you probably have other people available to help. If you're eighty-two and live alone, your social supports are likely to be much weaker. Although moving on to a rehab facility is rare for most patients, it is a very real alternative for older or physically disabled ones.

If you had atrial fibrillation or a wound infection after surgery and didn't panic, then you've experienced, in a very personal way, how to work through difficulty and continue to heal. Seen in this light, surgery can be a growth experience as well as a healing one.

Maybe you've adopted some new techniques for relaxation like massage, meditation, or music. Or you've dipped into some more familiar ones for support, like prayer and positive thinking. You are leaving the hospital a little bowed and broken, but with confidence that you can take over the reins of returning to strength and to your lifestyle. And maybe you've also learned that, instead of being rebuffed, when you are proactive and informed, you are more likely to get what you want.

It's very hard to quantify how much a feeling of serenity, or a prayer and a massage, can actually add to the scientific techniques of surgery and medicine. Patients often won't tell their doctors that they feel better about surgery because they know their church congregation is saying special prayers for them, or that a psychologist has taught them hypnosis to help them deal with anxiety about the operation.

Studies at Columbia Presbyterian have shown that while more than 70 percent of surgical patients there use some form of techniques that supplement the traditional medical ones, only 30 percent said they were willing to discuss it with their physicians. They are embarrassed, concerned the doctor doesn't know anything about the subject, and fearful of compromising the relationship with the doctor or offending her. Remember, however, that surgeons appreciate the benefits of working with a patient who has a healthy spiritual and psychological approach to surgery and recovery. And as your medical advisor, she wants to know everything about you, including what vitamins you're taking that may act as blood thinners, or what herbs you're using that might interact with medications she prescribes. She needs to know your activities so that her advice is based on your whole picture.

When patients first hear they need an operation, many say to the doctor, when will you be ready to do it? The doctors do surgery every day. The real question is when are you, the patient, ready? In this day and age, many operations have about a 98 percent success rate, including delicate heart surgeries. The battle isn't just to get you through the operation, but to get you to thrive after it.

If that battle gets too hard during recovery, speak to your doctor, psychologist, complementary-medicine practitioner, or a religious counselor. Even if you've had little challenge in the aftermath of surgery, remember to be kind to yourself instead of pushing to do more, faster.

You can work on envisioning a positive recovery period right from the first days of the diagnosis. And you can adopt an approach that works no matter what challenge comes up; be a proactive consumer who asks questions until the answers are clear and who makes the fullest use of the personal and medical resources available.

The hospital staff have been the facilitators, moving you on to the next stage of health and recovery. You've probably discovered that at no point along the way has it been better to abdicate total responsibility for your well-being to them. As much as you value the advice and skills of the medical professionals treating you, the possession of a medical education and a white coat does not mean that others have replaced you as the world's leading expert on your body.

If you weary of the challenge of staying informed and involved, remember a simple example. If a doctor is about to give you an injection and doesn't give you any warning, when she jabs you, it'll make you jump. You'll be even more fearful of her next move. On the other hand, if you know the prick is coming and why you're getting it, chances are that it simply won't hurt as much because you're expecting it.

There'll be moments in your surgical experience that feel like so many jabs in the arm. But you don't need to jump in pain or fear the next poke if you trust your medical team, agree with what they're doing and why they're doing it, and keep up your participation in choosing the best moves toward health and recovery.

There is one more step that will complete your preparation for surgery. You need to peek through the operating-room door and look at the details of the operation itself, which are covered in the following chapters.

10

What You Need to Know About Anesthesia

Mention the word *anesthesia* to a person older than forty, and chances are you'll get a shudder in response. I certainly sympathize. I'll never forget how I felt as a child getting anesthesia for an appendectomy. While I lay underneath a blinding bright light, the anesthetic dripped onto a gauze mask placed on my face. I had to breathe in this horrible-smelling stuff. That was about forty years ago, back in the days when the agent was ether, an anesthetic so flammable it could explode, and so variable in its effect, it actually induced a state of excitement before it put you to sleep.

Now fast-forward to today, when the anesthetic agents are high-quality and diverse, their dosages measured with extreme precision, and their delivery equipment as reliable as a jet engine. The progress since ether, the first widely available anesthetic, which had been in use since the mid-1800s, has been remarkable. Today no one uses ether, or any other agent that is flammable. The number of anesthetics continues to proliferate, and the ability to monitor the effect of those drugs has greatly improved.

And yet, some people still consider anesthesia a throwback to the dark ages. There's no need to put yourself through that anxiety. The way to deal with your concerns about anesthesia is to make sure you speak to an anesthesiologist in the days or weeks before your surgery. Find out the facts about anesthesia; get all your questions answered. Consider this visit vital both for you and the anesthesiologist.

The topic of anesthesia deserves your attention and your input. As one anesthesiologist put it, "Most people think my job is putting people to sleep. That's really inaccurate. What's most important is that I am able to wake patients up." There's a lot of wisdom in that.

MEETING THE ANESTHESIOLOGIST

You might not have "make an appointment with an anesthesiologist at the hospital" on your TO DO list. Don't wait for your surgeon to make the appointment for you; many don't bring it up as an option. There's no more important step you can take to learn what to expect from anesthesia.

In the old days, ten years ago or more, making a separate visit several days in advance of surgery to see an anesthesiologist wasn't necessary. That's when you checked into the hospital an entire day or two before the operation. There was plenty of time for the anesthesiologist to meet with you then and go over the next day's drill. Now, with managed-care policies and changes in technology, most patients arrive only hours before their surgery.

Where does that put the first contact between the anesthesiologist and you? Just minutes before the operation begins.

It's been clear throughout this book that you can put yourself in control of the process of surgery, right up to the time the surgeon takes over in the operating room. The way you do that is by meeting with the key medical personnel, asking questions, gathering data, and making informed choices among the available options.

That process does not work nearly so smoothly if you leave any important part of it, including an understanding of anesthesia, to the day of surgery. Some institutions make it easy for you. At Columbia-Presbyterian, there is an anesthesiology clinic available when you arrive for your pre-surgical tests. If there isn't a similar way to meet the anesthesiologist at your hospital, ask your surgeon for help in making the appointment in advance.

In an operation, the anesthesiologist is a very important part of the surgical team and works closely with the surgeon. Each hospital, and sometimes each department within that hospital, may have different policies on who chooses the anesthesiologist for a particular operation. For example, the surgeon may choose, or it may be based on a rotation system. The one you meet in a pre-surgical visit is likely to be different from the one who is in the operating room the day of your surgery, especially in a large hospital with many anesthesiologists on staff.

In any good hospital, all anesthesiologists should be board-certified. When medical personnel put you to sleep, you want them to have had their skills judged using the highest standards of the profession. You can rely on board certification as one good mechanism to identify competence. Nurse anesthetists may also perform anesthesia at some facilities, under the supervision of an attending anesthesiologist, and they also have a board-certification process.

When you meet with an anesthesiologist, you can discuss your concerns without the pressure of an imminent operation. Equally relevant, this discussion can uncover any information that the anesthesiologist needs to know. A patient may be in for a simple surgery, but what if she has other complex medical problems? Of course, the surgeon has considered these issues in the context of the operation; however, the anesthesiologist's particular skill is to evaluate their effect on the type and method of anesthesia. By meeting in advance, the chances of a surprise surfacing on the day of surgery are greatly reduced.

For example, the anesthesiologist may see a patient and decide there's a concern about the patient's heart. The prudent course would be to see a cardiologist before the operation. There's time to do that before the scheduled surgery. But if this observation is made the day of surgery, the operation may have to be canceled for that day. That's a frustrating result for everyone. In some cases, tests may not come back until just before the operation, or other new information may surface. You can't eliminate every possibility, but you can certainly pave the way for a safe and successful operation by a simple visit beforehand.

It might seem obvious to meet the anesthesiologist early on if you're having a complex surgery or if you have other serious medical problems. But what if you're eighteen years old and having your tonsils out? Ask any anesthesiologist what she would do if it were her child, and what you'll most likely hear is, "Yes, I'd have the meeting."

Whether or not you speak with an anesthesiologist in advance, on the day of your surgery you will meet the anesthesiologist who will administer anesthesia to you and be present in the operating room. All discussions and results of tests will be reviewed and finalized at that point.

TYPES OF ANESTHESIA

In a typical surgery, it takes between ten and twenty minutes from the time a patient is anesthetized to when the first incision is made. Often the process starts with the patient receiving a mild sedative and medication to dry up secretions in the mouth and other passages. It ends when you wake up, which in most operations is in the operating room or in some cases, in the intensive-care unit.

Depending on the institution, the preparation for surgery is done in a holding area outside the actual operating room or in the OR itself. The part of the body to be operated on is thoroughly cleansed to disinfect it, shaved if necessary, and draped with sterile cloth.

The patient has one or more catheters placed in veins to make it possible to introduce intravenous fluids, including anesthetic drugs, during surgery on a continuous basis. The patient is also attached to several monitors that are essential for measuring signs such as blood pressure, heart rate, and amount of oxygen.

When there is a choice of anesthesia, it is between local and/or regional anesthesia and general. One of the most familiar scenarios for choosing anesthesia is childbirth. A woman's options include oral pain medication, spinal injection, general anesthesia, or nothing at all.

Or, if a patient is having knee surgery and is otherwise healthy, it may make no significant difference in risk factors if the patient has local or general anesthesia. However, if the patient has very bad asthma, the anesthesiologist might advise a spinal because general anesthesia could exacerbate the asthma.

In other procedures, such as open-heart or lung surgery, there is no choice. A patient must have general anesthesia in order to stay immobilized.

Patients' predilections vary tremendously. Some say, "Put me to sleep, I don't want to know anything." (Remember my earlier references to autonomy dumping?) Others look forward to being not only aware and awake, but able to watch the operation on a television monitor, which is possible in some kinds of endoscopic surgery.

Whichever end of the spectrum you fall on, it helps to understand the various types of anesthesia and what is happening in your body when they are introduced.

General

General anesthesia is usually administered intravenously, although in some cases inhalation gases are used. It provides the following effects:

- Analgesia: no pain during surgery.

- Sedation: no awareness during surgery.

- Amnesia: no memory of the surgery.

- Immobility: no movement during surgery.

The amount of pain relief, sedation, and paralysis varies with the individual patient and the type of surgery. In open-heart surgery, for example, deep anesthesia is required. Paralysis must be complete, and the patient has to have a breathing tube inserted, which allows breathing to take place through a ventilator.

The experience of general anesthesia is likened to the deepest sleep—you are totally unaware of what's happening. And, just like a deep sleep, you can be roused out of it. In this case, you won't wake up until the anesthesiologist is ready to wake you up, a process that is slow and gradual. You will be groggy, not completely "with it," and unable to remember what just happened. But you will be awake and able to move when the anesthesiologist withdraws the anesthetic agents.

Local and/or Regional Anesthesia

In local anesthesia, the tissues or peripheral nerves at the actual site of the surgery are numbed, usually by injection, though topical anesthetics may also be used.

In regional anesthesia, a nerve block numbs the nerves at some distance from the site of surgery. It prevents a person from feeling anything in the area controlled by those nerves. The most common is a spinal or an epidural, an injection of an anesthetic into the fluid around the spine or into the epidural space in the back. In hand surgery, for example, the nerve block may be injected into the arm.

In some cases, the anesthesiologist will give a combination of a regional and local injection. This is often done at the end of the operation to help with pain as the patient is easing off the regional nerve block.

Usually the patient is sedated with a separate medication. Calming medication helps you deal with any anxiety or discomfort. It's difficult to lie on a table in full awareness of the sights and sounds of an operating room without getting at least a little agitated. Also, even though the nerve block prevents pain, there may be a sensation of pressure on the area being treated. The sedation is short-acting and may be Valium, a narcotic, or a hypnotic drug. A person is not likely to feel groggy from it after the operation. Of course, you can choose to forego sedation.

FEARS

There are many fears surrounding anesthesia. No matter how far-fetched they sound to you, do not be embarrassed to raise them.

All drugs have side effects and those that anesthetize you are no exception. Nausea and vomiting, low blood pressure, headaches after a spinal, or sore throat from a breathing tube are a few of them. Beyond these, certain drugs may have a particular effect because of your state of health. Some anesthetics are metabolized and excreted through the kidneys. If a patient is suffering from kidney failure, those drugs would not be used to anesthetize that patient.

You need to find out what side effects are relevant in your particular case. And you need to distinguish reasonable concerns from irrational fears stemming from misconceptions, complications that are extremely rare, or problems that are no longer an issue due to contemporary drugs, equipment, and monitoring.

Some patients tell me, "My grandmother had anesthesia and it sounded barbaric." It probably was barbaric. But that was then and this is now. The major questions are, "Am I going to feel pain?" and "Am I going to wake up?" Once you get these questions resolved by a qualified anesthesiologist, express what else is on your mind. I've heard all these topics raised at one time or another:

Paralysis During General Anesthesia

Paralysis can be a frightening thought and you should raise it if you have any concerns about what that means in relation to anesthesia.

Have you heard tales of a patient under general anesthesia who feels pain, but can't tell anyone because the anesthesia makes a patient unable to speak or move a finger?

This would be an extremely rare occurrence. You can counter this worry with your trust in a highly competent anesthesiologist who knows just what dosages to give you. Backing her up is a set of very reliable equipment whose monitoring capability would signal a problem.

If you are feeling pain, your vital signs speak for you, like rapid heart rate and rising blood pressure. Your anesthesiologist continuously monitors them, and during surgery and at any sign of a problem, medication can be immediately adjusted through the IV already in place.

Paralysis from Spinal Anesthesia

Some people will say, "Don't give me a spinal. My mother knew someone who was paralyzed from it." That may have happened in the past, but new equipment has changed that risk. Until the mid-1970s, spinal anesthesia was delivered by a needle that had been used, then washed in alcohol. The problem was that alcohol can be very damaging to nerves and occasionally a patient became paralyzed, not from the anesthetic, but from the method of cleaning the needle. Now the needle has a disposable tip; it's used, then thrown out, and alcohol is not introduced into spinal fluid.

Fear of Not Waking Up

The anesthetic drugs are not irreversibly toxic. If there is some form of brain injury that prevents a person from waking up, it is likely to be due to a lack of oxygen to the brain. That's why most instances of general anesthesia are accompanied by the insertion of a breathing tube to ensure by mechanical means that an adequate supply of oxygen is going to the body at all times during surgery. When the diaphragm is paralyzed, this allows the anesthesiologist to take complete control over your breathing. If this lack of control over your own breathing frightens you, remember that the systems and equipment for doing the breathing for you are remarkably sophisticated.

Concerns About Your Behavior While Under Local or Regional Anesthesia

Are you afraid if you have local or regional anesthesia that you will move and cause the surgeon to cut in the wrong place? You should expect to get the kind of information and support from the medical team so that you are positioned properly and will not move in a potentially damaging way. At Columbia Presbyterian there is a surgeon who is one of the few in the country who performs delicate thyroid and parathyroid surgery in the neck under local anesthesia. Patients keep still with the help of careful instructions from the surgeon. In addition, sedation keeps you from moving around during surgery.

General Anxiety

Usually, the anxieties of a patient are diminished when he has been fully informed about anesthesia in advance of surgery, and sedated just before the operation. Relaxation techniques, like soothing tapes, can also help.

But some patients suffer from a recognized psychiatric condition called panic disorder. They may experience extraordinary feelings of terror about the operation from the time they hear a diagnosis right up to when they arrive to check in for surgery. They may be so panicked they just don't show up, in which case it's necessary to cancel the operation. Unless the surgery is an emergency, it can be post-poned until a patient can treat the disorder, often with drugs called beta-blockers. Once a patient is on beta blockers, the anesthesiologist takes this into account in deciding the best anesthetic agents to use during surgery.

———

The anesthesiologist does far more than inject you with an agent. She is there for the entire surgery, watching you, making sure your blood pressure, heart rate, and breathing are normal and that there is adequate oxygenation of your blood. She is checking that your depth of anesthesia is appropriate, and you're not feeling anything or moving around. She will make sure you wake up, and when you do, that you will not have a lot of pain.

In earlier chapters, we discussed the issues of information and trust. Once again, you need to feel confident you can place your trust in a qualified anesthesiologist who is part of a highly competent medical team bolstered by state-of-the-art equipment.

Part Three

WHAT'S GOING
TO HAPPEN
TO ME?

11

A Brief Introduction to the Surgical Procedures

To help you understand the surgery you are considering, the following chapters detail forty-five of the most common surgeries, accompanied by illustrations. This is no substitute for having a qualified physician evaluate your individual state of health, and your options for treating the specific problem. The overview of each surgery tells you in general terms what the issues are and what is likely to happen. It is a framework of basic knowledge and a springboard for your questions.

The procedures are organized alphabetically within nine systems of the body (e.g., orthopedic) or types of surgery (transplants). The procedures are grouped in chapters that explain the surgery for:

Cancer operations to treat cancer of the breast and skin.
Cardiothoracic operations on the heart and lungs.
Endocrine operations on organs that secrete hormones.
Gastrointestinal operations that involve the digestive system, including the colon, pancreas, and esophagus.
General procedures that are very common and not categorizable as part of another classification.
Orthopedic surgery on the bones and joints of the body.
Reproductive operations on organs that enable pregnancy.
Transplantation operations including heart, lung, and kidney transplants.
Vascular surgery that involves the blood vessels.

Information for each surgery is divided as follows:

Definition and Part of Body Operated On

These descriptions tell you just what the surgery does and identify what area or organ is being operated on. In some cases, more detail is provided to explain complicated anatomy.

Reasons for Having the Operation

The typical symptoms or problems that make it necessary to view surgery as an option.

What Could Happen if You Don't Have the Operation

In some cases you could do nothing or use medication to relieve symptoms; in others, the condition could lead to death. You need to know where on this spectrum your problem lies.

*Factors That Increase Your Risk of Complications**

There are certain medical or lifestyle conditions that could make it more likely that you'll have problems during or after surgery. Typically, poor general health, serious heart or respiratory ailments, and negative habits like smoking may make it harder to have a smooth operation and recovery.

Although I don't list your surgeon's skill, it is certainly another factor affecting your risk. You are far more likely to get the result you want with a surgeon who is highly experienced in the specific type of surgery you are having. Do not hesitate to find out how many operations exactly like yours your surgeon has actually done. As new techniques become popular, this is particularly important. If you have a choice between endoscopic and open surgery, for example, the quicker recovery and smaller incisions of endoscopic

---

*The entries in these categories have been organized alphabetically.

surgery may sway your decision. But you have to factor in the issues of limited visibility and surgical experience.

Possible Complications During and After Surgery*

In most surgeries, bleeding and infection are possible, if unlikely, complications. In addition, each surgery has its own set of complications that could occur.

Tests You May Have to Undergo*

Any reputable institution has policies about pre-surgical testing which generally include blood tests, and depending on age and condition, chest X rays and EKGs. Beyond that, most surgeries have a specific set of tests to confirm the diagnosis and clarify decisions about the operation.

Basic Steps of the Operation

This is a brief overview in simple, nontechnical language so that you, as a patient, will know what is being done to your body during surgery. In certain cases, the description is the very latest in that particular type of surgery, so it might not describe exactly how your surgeon will perform the operation. The accompanying illustrations either depict the entire procedure or highlight a key aspect of a more complex operation.

What to Expect When It's Over

There are general results you can expect in terms of pain, recovery time, and care in the days or weeks following surgery. This will help you understand whether you'll be out of work for a week or three months and some of the sensations or difficulties you may experience as you return to normal life activities. Remember always that pain and recovery experiences are very individualized.

---

*The entries in these categories have been organized alphabetically.

If you have read this book and followed its recommendations, there is one result you can expect, no matter what your condition and your type of surgery. You can go through the operation and its recovery with the knowledge that you have done all that you possibly could to make the experience and the outcome a positive one for your health.

12

Breast and Skin Cancer Surgery

BREAST LUMPECTOMY

After a tumor or abnormal mass in the breast has been diag-
nosed as malignant, a lumpectomy may be done to remove the
malignancy and its surrounding tissue. Additionally, the sur-
geon usually removes some of the lymph nodes under the arm
to check for cancer. (The term excisional biopsy *describes a*
procedure in which the lesion is removed, but a cancer diag-
nosis is not certain pre-operatively, and a margin of normal
tissue around the lesion may not be included.)

Part of the body operated on:
The breast; possibly the armpit.

Reasons for having the operation:
To remove a malignant mass in the breast that has been discovered
either by touch in a physical exam or through a mammogram, ultrasound, or other breast-imaging technique.

What could happen if you don't have the operation:
The cancer could spread to other organs and become life-threatening.
The breast cancer itself could progress locally to an advanced stage,
causing pain, skin changes, ulceration, and bleeding from the breast.

Factors that increase your risk of complications:
Bleeding disorders or use of anticlotting therapies that could increase the risk of post-operative bleeding.
Impaired immune function that could lead to infection.
Poor health due to other serious medical conditions.

Possible complications during and after surgery:
A lumpectomy is generally a low-risk operation and complications are rare. Less than 1 percent of patients experience bleeding or infection after surgery.

Tests you may have to undergo:
Blood tests.
A bone scan may be recommended if the lumpectomy is being performed for a cancer above a certain size.
Chest X ray.
EKG.

Basic steps of the operation:
1. The patient is positioned on the operating table in a supine position and is sedated.
2. The breast is cleansed with an antiseptic solution and local anesthesia is injected into the area where the surgery will be done.

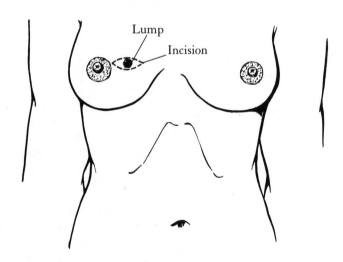

3. A skin incision is made in the anesthetized area directly over the mass.
4. Scissors or scalpel are used to delineate and dissect the area of breast tissue being removed, which includes the entire abnormality, plus a margin of surrounding tissue.
5. The tissue that is removed is marked in such a way that the examining pathologist can assess the edges of the tissue and understand the tissue's orientation within the breast.
6. The surgical area is inspected for other abnormalities.
7. Any bleeding vessels are controlled using a cautery device. The area is irrigated with saline solution.
8. If an axillary lymph-node procedure is being done at the same time, a small incision is made in the armpit and some of the lymph nodes are removed.
9. The skin is closed using absorbable sutures under the skin. A dressing is applied.

Duration: 30 minutes.

What to expect when it's over:
The recovery period is generally brief, about 24 to 48 hours.

Putting an ice pack on the area that was cut during the first 12 hours after surgery decreases pain and swelling. Oral medication is prescribed for pain control.

Wearing a bra, even at night, is helpful for the first few days.

Vigorous exercise involving the upper body should be avoided for at least 1 week after surgery in order to avoid interfering with wound healing.

When the pathology report is available, the doctor will discuss the results and formulate a treatment plan. That may include radiation to reduce chances of recurrence, chemotherapy if cancer is found in the lymph nodes, a mastectomy, or a combination of therapies.

BREAST RECONSTRUCTION

Creating a new breast for a woman after her own is removed, usually because of breast cancer. The woman's own tissue or an implant may be used for the reconstruction.

Part of the body operated on:
The breast.
The abdomen (the back, rarely, if body tissue is being used).

Reasons for having the operation:
When a patient has a mastectomy, she has the option to have no reconstruction, do reconstruction during the mastectomy, or delay it.

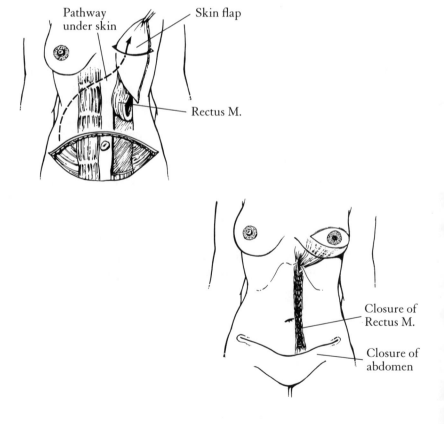

Considerations for making the decision of when to have the surgery and what method to use include the following:

Immediate reconstruction avoids the need for another operation at a later date, but it adds time to the 2-hour mastectomy surgery—about an hour for an implant, about 4 hours for using body tissue. It may also increase the risk of complications and the amount of recovery time.

The implant requires a second procedure several months later to replace the temporary implant with a permanent one.

If a patient uses her own tissue, when she wakes up after a mastectomy, she will have a reconstructed breast. The implant is not fully inflated until several months later.

The use of tissue may result in a breast that looks more natural; an implant may not hang as normally as the other breast, though it will look nearly the same in a bra.

Surgery using tissue is more major than that of an implant and more extensive than a mastectomy.

In either case, patients also have the option of doing a procedure on the other breast to make it more symmetrical with the reconstructed breast, including breast reduction, lift, or augmentation.

What could happen if you don't have the operation:
A patient would have a flat chest on the side where the breast was removed.

Factors that increase your risk of complications:
Other serious medical problems (diabetes, heart disease).
For some, but not all, types of reconstruction, previous radiation therapy and obesity are risk factors.
Smoking.

Possible complications during and after surgery:
Bleeding.
Infection.
Unsightly scarring.
If abdominal tissue is used: hernia or abdominal bulge.
If an implant is used: implant deflation or collapse, extrusion or pushing out, distortion.

Tests you may have to undergo:
Blood tests (blood count, electrolytes, coagulation).
Chest X ray.
EKG.

Basic steps of the operation:
Reconstruction using the patient's own tissue:

1. Abdominal tissue, called a TRAM flap, is the most common source of tissue for a new breast. Scars created by the removal of tissue are generally well concealed in the abdomen and since the tissue that is used would normally be discarded in an operation that reduces the abdomen, the patient is in effect getting a tummy tuck.

2. A long horizontal incision is made from one side of the abdomen to the other above the pubic area. A large ellipse of tissue is cut from mostly below the belly button. The tissue that's been cut is left attached to the underlying muscle and blood supply.

3. The surgeon makes a tunnel deep in the fat from the abdomen up to the breast. The tissue is then pulled up through the tunnel, rotated into its new position in the chest, and reshaped into a breast.

4. In some cases, the tissue for reconstruction may be removed completely from the underlying tissue and then must be reattached in the chest area using microsurgery.

Duration: 4 hours.

For a reconstruction using an implant:

1. A breast expander (a balloonlike device made from silicone rubber) is placed in a deflated state under the tissue that remains from the breast that's been removed.

2. For several months thereafter, the patient goes to the doctor's office for repeated injections of small amounts of sterile saline (salt water) by means of a small needle through the skin. The saline gradually expands the device and the tissue over it begins to stretch. This creates a breast-shaped pocket for a breast implant. A patient may feel pressure or discomfort, which subsides as the tissue expands.

3. When the expander has been inflated to the desired size, there is a second outpatient procedure (often under local anesthesia

and intravenous sedation, though it may also be done under general anesthesia). The expander is removed and replaced in the pocket with a permanent implant that is an unfilled silicone rubber shell. The shell is then filled with a saline solution. *Duration: 2 hours.*

Several months after reconstruction is complete in either procedure and the swelling in the reconstructed breast has gone down, the nipple and areola are reconstructed in the doctor's office under local anesthesia. The nipple is reconstructed with flaps of skin at the site, and the nipple and areola are tattooed to the appropriate color. Occasionally, skin grafts may be used in the procedure.

What to expect when it's over:
If a patient's tissue is used, she remains in the hospital for about 4 days. When an expander is placed, hospitalization is slightly shorter. Patients are usually walking by the second day. Narcotic pain medication is administered through patient-controlled pumps until the pain is reduced and patients can take pain relief orally. Recovery is about 1 to 2 weeks with an expander/implant; about 3 to 4 weeks if abdominal tissue is used.

MASTECTOMY/BREAST REMOVAL

Simple (total) mastectomy: *removal of the entire breast.*
Modified radical mastectomy: *removal of the entire breast along with the lymph nodes under the armpit.*
Radical mastectomy: *removal of the breast, the lymph nodes, chest muscles, and additional fat and skin. This operation is very rarely done today.*

Part of the body operated on:
The breast and the armpit.

Reasons for having the operation:
To remove a cancerous breast, or as a prophylactic (infrequently done). Some women at high risk for breast cancer may choose to re-move a breast, after reviewing other options that include careful monitoring and medication, to prevent the future development of breast cancer.

What could happen if you don't have the operation:
For early-stage breast cancer, the best surgical option is to remove the tumor and surrounding tissue and armpit lymph nodes (breast

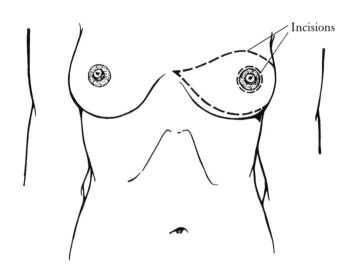

Incisions

conservation or lumpectomy). If the cancer is untreated, it could spread and cause death.

Factors that increase your risk of complications:
Bleeding problems.
Diabetes.
Heart or lung disease, or poor overall health.
Smoking.

Possible complications during and after surgery:
Accumulation of fluid at the site of the operation (seroma).
Bleeding.
Infection.
Swollen arm (lymphedema), decreased sensation in upper inner arm, decreased range of motion and strength.

Tests you may have to undergo:
Biopsy (removal of cells or tissue from the breast for diagnosis).
Blood tests.
Chest X ray.
EKG.
Mammography (breast-imaging by low-dose X ray).

Basic steps of the operation:
1. The patient is administered general anesthesia.
2. An incision is made around the nipple and areola and at the site of the biopsy. The incision may extend out to the armpit.
3. The breast tissue is removed; as much skin as possible is preserved.
4. Some of the lymph nodes in the armpit are removed. The extent of the removal is discussed with the surgeon prior to the operation.
5. One or more drainage tubes are inserted into the area where the nodes and/or the breast tissue were removed.
6. Breast reconstruction may be performed at this time, if chosen by the patient pre-operatively. If so, surgery would continue. (See Breast Reconstruction on page 170.)
7. If there is no reconstruction, the incision is closed with sutures.
Duration: 2 hours.

What to expect when it's over:

One to 2 nights in the hospital; longer with certain types of reconstruction.

Physical therapy to restore arm strength and range of motion and to counter temporary tightness in the breast area and stiffness in the arm and shoulder.

If the patient has a drainage tube (or tubes) in her wound, she must care for it at home by emptying the tube and recording the volume of fluid every day. This usually lasts about 1 week, but in some cases could be several weeks. Once the fluid level has decreased enough to remove the tube, the patient must return to the surgeon's office to have it done.

Patients generally feel better within 2 weeks; full recovery takes about 4 to 6 weeks.

Patients may require continuing treatment with radiation or chemotherapy.

Many women find it very difficult after surgery to deal with the loss of a breast. Patients are encouraged to join a support group of other women who have had mastectomies and/or pursue one-on-one counseling with a qualified therapist.

MELANOMA/SKIN LESION REMOVAL

This operation removes a cancerous skin lesion and an area of surrounding tissue called the margin. There are three types of skin cancer. Basal cell *cancer is the least invasive with the least amount of margin removed;* squamous cell *is more aggressive with a wider margin required.* Melanoma *is the most serious type of skin cancer, occurring in the cells that produce pigment.*

Many types of benign skin growths may look like malignant tumors and are removed for a biopsy. If a lesion looks precancerous it may be removed as a precaution.

Part of the body operated on:
The skin on any part of the body where the lesion is located.

Reasons for having the operation:
To remove a cancerous tumor and prevent it from growing.

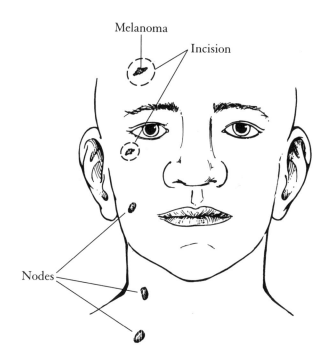

Melanoma

Incision

Nodes

What could happen if you don't have the operation:
The cancer could enlarge locally and/or spread to other parts of the body.

Factors that increase your risk of complications:
Diabetes.
Heart disease.

Possible complications during and after surgery:
Bleeding.
Infection.

Tests you may have to undergo:
Biopsy.
Blood tests.
X rays.

Basic steps of the operation:
1. Anesthesia may be general or local.
2. An incision is made at the site of the cancer. The size of the incision depends on the size and depth of the lesion.
3. In some cases, a frozen section is done. Tissue is removed for biopsy and analyzed immediately by a pathologist. If it is cancerous, the entire lesion is removed while the patient is still anesthetized.
4. Some types of tumors are not conducive to a frozen section. In those cases, a biopsy is done first on a suspicious growth. A full pathology report is prepared, and if the growth is cancerous, then the entire area is removed in an operation performed at a later date.
5. Surrounding tissue is removed. The amount depends on the type of tumor, its depth, and level of penetration.
6. Nearby lymph nodes may also removed. Very early cancers can generally be removed without the lymph nodes.
7. When the growth path of advanced melanomas is difficult to detect, a process called *scintillography* may be performed. A radioactive dye is injected into the site of the malignancy and tracked by a medical instrument similar to a Geiger counter.

By determining the direction that the dye drains from the site, the surgeon identifies the likely path of the tumor's growth and removes that tissue as well as the nearby lymph nodes.

8. The surgeon closes the incision with sutures, tucking them as much as possible in the folds and creases of the skin to minimize visibility. If the incision is too large for suturing, a skin graft or skin flap (adjacent tissue) may be used instead.

Duration: 1½ hours with nodes, unless skin graft needed.

What to expect when it's over:

The surgery is usually done on an outpatient basis, unless a skin graft is necessary.

The incision requires minimal care and normal activities, with the exception of vigorous exercise, can be quickly resumed.

Pain is generally controlled by oral medication.

13

Cardiothoracic Surgery

BALLOON ANGIOPLASTY OR CORONARY STENTING

A catheter tube with a balloon at its tip is placed at the site of a blockage in a coronary artery. The balloon is inflated for a short period of time and then deflated to open the artery and permit blood to flow more freely. In most patients, a coronary stent (metal scaffolding) is then inserted at the site of the blockage.

Part of the body operated on:
Coronary arteries.

Reasons for having the operation:
Pain or heaviness in the chest on exertion to a blockage in the coronary artery (stable exertional angina).
Abnormal exercise stress test due to a blocked artery (silent ischemia).
Chest pain at rest or during minimal exertion (unstable angina).
To open up a completely blocked coronary artery within the first 6 hours of a heart attack. This is called primary balloon angioplasty and primary coronary stenting.

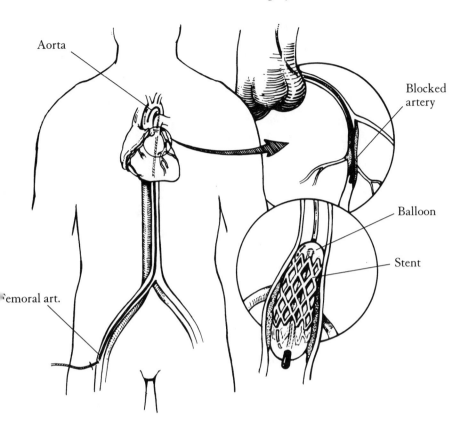

What could happen if you don't have the operation:
A coronary artery that is completely blocked and/or a heart attack, which damages muscle, or causes death.

Factors that increase your risk of complications:
Bleeding diathesis (prolonged bleeding after an injury).
Congestive heart failure (the heart is unable to pump the necessary volume of blood).
Diabetes.
Renal failure (reduction in the ability of the kidneys to filter and excrete waste products).
Severe peripheral vascular disease (narrowing of the blood vessels in the legs and arms resulting in restricted blood flow).

Possible complications during and after surgery:
Arrhythmia (abnormal rhythm or rate of heartbeat).
Bleeding.
Death (extremely rare).
Heart attack.
In less than 1 percent of patients, the coronary artery abruptly closes, which in rare cases leads to emergency coronary artery bypass surgery.
Infection.
Kidney failure.
Stroke.
Vascular complications in the arm or leg at the site of the insertion of the tube.

Tests you may have to undergo:
Cardiac catheterization.
Stress tests (not in all cases).

Basic steps of the operation:
1. The patient's groin (or in some cases, the arm) is draped, prepped, and anesthetized with local anesthesia.
2. Two tubes or sheaths are placed into the femoral artery and vein in the leg. A guiding catheter (tube) is inserted through the sheath in the femoral artery and advanced backward through the aorta to the opening of the diseased coronary artery.
3. The guiding catheter is then inserted into the opening of the coronary artery and contrast dye is used to see the diseased artery via X ray.
4. A guidewire (thin wire) is inserted through the guiding catheter and into the diseased coronary artery, through the tight blockage, and into the farther end of the coronary artery.
5. The balloon catheter (tube with a balloon at its tip) is advanced over the wire to the site of the blockage and inflated for about 60 seconds, two or three times, followed by deflation to open up the blockage. The balloon is removed.
6. In about 80 percent of the patients, a coronary artery stent (metal scaffolding) is inserted at the site of the blockage. The

stent is delivered on a balloon that is then inflated, opening the stent and apposing the metal struts to the wall of the coronary artery. The use of the stent results in a much smaller rate of re-narrowing of the artery than by balloon angioplasty alone.

7. The guidewire, balloon catheter, and guiding catheter are removed from the body. The sheaths in the femoral artery and vein are temporarily sewn in. They are removed a few hours later (up to 12 hours).

8. The patient lies flat on his back during the entire procedure and for at least 8 hours after the sheaths have been removed to make sure there is no bleeding from the femoral artery or vein (both large vessels).

Duration: 2 to 3 hours.

What to expect when it's over:

A patient is usually discharged within 24 to 48 hours.

He must take an aspirin a day indefinitely. If he had a stent put in place, he remains on the aspirin permanently. He also takes an additional oral blood thinner for the first 2 to 4 weeks after the procedure to prevent the metallic stent from clotting; he should not have an MRI for at least 8 weeks after the procedure.

A patient can usually return to work within 1 week of the procedure.

Both balloon angioplasty and coronary artery stenting have a greater than 95 percent initial success rate in opening up blockages.

There is a 30 to 40 percent chance that a coronary artery will renarrow (restenosis) at the site of balloon angioplasty within the first 3 to 6 months after the procedure. However, there is only a 10 to 20 percent chance that it will renarrow if a coronary stent has been placed at the site.

BRONCHOSCOPY

The insertion of a bronchoscope (a flexible, lighted tube) through the nose and down the trachea (the windpipe) and into the lungs. The tube is equipped with a lens and instruments that enable the surgeon to see into the bronchi, the main airways in the lungs, and to treat various conditions. If a patient is having surgery or is on a ventilator (breathing machine), he may already have another tube, called an endotracheal tube, in place in his windpipe. In that case, the bronchoscope goes down the endotracheal tube.

Part of the body operated on:
The lungs, accessed by going through the larynx, trachea, and bronchi.

Reasons for having the operation:
To determine the nature of various lung conditions:

Nodules (small lumps of tissue).
Tumors (abnormal masses of tissue that are biopsied for cancer).
Fibrous tissue (scar or connective tissue).
Pneumonia (inflammation of the lungs from infection).

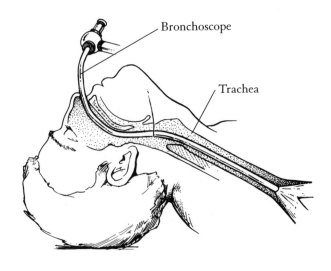

Bronchoscope

Trachea

To relieve obstruction by removing mucus (thick, slimy liquid) or foreign bodies.

What could happen if you don't have the operation:
Failure to diagnose and treat a problem like cancer.
Suffocation from presence of foreign matter in the lungs.

Factors that increase your risk of complications:
Bleeding disorders.
Negative health and lifestyle habits like smoking, alcoholism, or drug abuse.
Recent illness of infection.
Respiratory distress.

Possible complications during and after surgery:
Bleeding. If bleeding does occur, it is almost always minimal and self-limiting. Significant bleeding is a very rare complication of bronchoscopic biopsies, occurring in less than 1 percent of cases.
Pneumothorax (lung collapse). This is a rare complication (occurring in less than 1 percent of cases) that results from a puncture of the lung during biopsies across the bronchi. It usually improves on its own. In a small number of cases, a tube needs to be inserted through the wall of the chest to re-expand the lung.

Tests you may have to undergo:
Blood tests, including coagulation (clotting studies).
CT scan (cross-sectional images of the body produced by scanning with an X ray and computer).
X rays.

Basic steps of the operation:
When a doctor is doing this procedure to diagnose a condition (a diagnostic bronch), it is usually done on an outpatient basis; when a therapeutic bronch (i.e., section, removal of foreign body, placement of stent, or removal of a growth) is done, it is often necessary to stay in the hospital.

1. The patient is generally awake during the procedure. He is given medication to control coughing and to induce relaxation.

A local anesthetic is used to numb the nose and the throat and allow the tube to be passed through them. The patient breathes on his own with oxygen through a mask and then a broncho-scope.

2. The surgeon inserts the tube and manipulates it to view the bronchial tree.

3. Instruments attached to the bronchoscope enable the surgeon to collect mucus, remove tissues for biopsy, and cut out growths or foreign bodies.

4. A bronchoscope is mainly used to examine and treat the bronchial tubes; in some cases, it may be used to examine the larynx and the trachea but treatments of those areas are usually done by other means, including a *laryngoscope*.

Duration: 30 to 45 minutes.

What to expect when it's over:
There is usually no discomfort after the procedure.
Some patients will have a mild sore throat.
The patient can eat in about 3 hours.
Results of some tests may be apparent immediately.
Biopsies or cultures may take several days or weeks for a final result.

CORONARY ARTERY BYPASS

This operation is done to bypass blockages in the coronary arteries that are restricting the flow of blood and oxygen to the heart. An artery from the chest and/or veins removed from the legs are grafted onto the heart and the coronary arteries, bypassing the blockage. The blood flow is rerouted through the newly created pathways.

Part of the body operated on:
Chest.
Legs.

Reasons for having the operation:
To avoid heart attack; to preserve heart function.

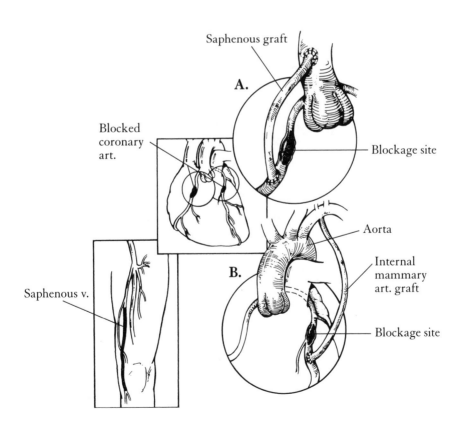

To prolong life by supplying the heart with adequate blood in patients with coronary artery disease.
To relieve symptoms of angina (chest, arm, neck, or abdominal pain due to improper blood supply to the heart).

What could happen if you don't have the operation:
Increased risk of heart attack, heart failure, and death.
Continued symptoms of angina.

Factors that increase your risk of complications:
Advanced age.
Diabetes.
Kidney failure.
Obesity.
Other forms of heart disease.
Smoking.

Possible complications during and after surgery:
Arrhythmia (irregular heartbeat; usually temporary).
Bleeding.
Death.
Heart attack.
Nerve injury to the hand/fingers (usually temporary).
Stroke.
Wound infection.

Tests you may have to undergo:
To determine need for a bypass:

Angiogram (the blood flow in vessels is made visible by an injected dye and projected on X-ray film).
EKG (recording electrical impulses of the heart), echocardiogram (images of the heart and its vessels through ultrasound), or a PET scan (a cross-sectional image of tissue activity by injection of a radioactive substance that is detected by sensors).
Stress test.

To determine fitness for surgery:
Blood tests.
Chest X ray.

EKG.

Urine tests.

Basic steps of the operation:

1. General anesthesia is administered; the chest and legs are cleansed and prepped for surgery.
2. An incision is made in the middle of the chest. The breastbone is divided with a saw.
3. The heart and aorta are exposed and are connected via tubing to a heart-lung machine, which takes over the functions of the heart and lungs while the heart is stopped.
4. Simultaneously, incisions are made in the legs and a length of vein is removed. An artery (internal mammary artery) in the chest is also isolated.
5. The blocked coronary artery is identified and an incision is made in it; one end of the vein from the leg is sewn to the opening in the artery; the other end is sewn to the aorta. If there is more than one blocked artery, this procedure is done for each one. The chest artery is sewn to a coronary artery and left attached at its origin.
6. Once the bypasses are in place, the heart is restarted. When it is beating well enough on its own, the heart-lung machine is removed.
7. Drainage tubes are placed in the chest to drain blood and air from around the heart and lungs. (They are removed in 1 to 2 days.)
8. The breastbone is closed with stainless-steel wires, the tissues above it are closed in layers, and the skin is closed with absorbable sutures.

Duration: 5 hours.

What to expect when it's over:

The patient will be in the intensive-care unit (ICU) for 1 to 2 days; the total hospital stay is about 5 to 7 days.

When the patient wakes up, there will be a breathing tube in his throat, which is removed when the patient is able to breathe well enough on his own, usually during the evening of the operation or the next morning.

By the second day, the patient usually is out of bed and walking.

Most patients have some pain, which can feel worse when coughing, sneezing, or laughing. Patient-controlled intravenous narcotic medications treat the pain; by the third or fourth day, generally only acetaminophen (Tylenol) is required for pain control.

By the time he leaves the hospital, the patient is able to walk stairs. At home, the patient can shower. Driving or lifting is not allowed for about 6 weeks while the breastbone heals.

Most normal activities can be resumed by 6 weeks, although the patient may experience fatigue on exertion. It takes about 3 to 6 months to return to full normalcy.

Patients should not smoke and should keep blood pressure, sugar level, and cholesterol under control.

Most or all of the angina should be relieved. Studies show that in 5 to 10 years, about a third of patients develop angina, which can be treated by medication, other procedures for the heart, or another bypass.

ELECTROPHYSIOLOGY (EP) STUDY/RADIOFREQUENCY ABLATION

An EP study assesses arrhythmias (abnormal heart rhythms) by inserting electrode catheters through the veins and into the heart; radiofrequency or catheter ablation destroys the parts of the electrical pathway that are causing the rapid heart rhythm. It is often done along with the EP study.

Part of the body operated on:
The heart. Insertion of the catheters takes place in the groin or, in some cases, the arm, chest, or neck.

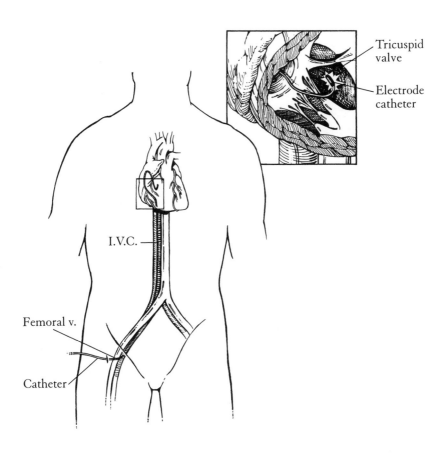

Tricuspid valve

Electrode catheter

I.V.C.

Femoral v.

Catheter

Reasons for having the operation:
Patient suffers from recurrent fast heart rhythms that interfere with daily activities and the condition is not improved by medication; in some cases the abnormal heartbeat is too slow.
The abnormal rhythms are severe enough to be life-threatening.
Patient has persistent symptoms of arrhythmia, but other means of testing have not been able to detect its location in the heart.
The EP study can record electrical signals, pace the heart by electrical impulses, or test medication while the arrhythmia is in process and being monitored. The catheter ablation is done if, once the cardiologist finds the source of the irregular beat, he determines that destroying it through heat is the best alternative.

What could happen if you don't have the operation:
Continued abnormal heart rhythms.
Palpitations, lightheadedness, fainting, chest pain, shortness of breath.
Serious impairment in the heart's ability to pump blood, which could cause death.

Factors that increase your risk of complications:
Advanced age.
Congestive heart failure.
Previous stroke.

Possible complications during and after surgery:
Bleeding at the site of catheter insertion; swelling or bruises.
Blood clots.
Damage to the heart or blood vessels.
Infection.

Tests you may have to undergo:
Blood tests.
EKG.

Basic steps of the operation:
1. The site where catheters are inserted is shaved and cleansed.
2. Patient is given a local anesthetic and sedation.

3. A small incision is made in the skin (usually the groin). A needle punctures the vein or artery into which a catheter is inserted.
4. One or more electrode catheters (long flexible wires that can conduct electrical impulses to and from the heart) are threaded to the heart and positioned inside it, close to the abnormal electrical pathway.
5. The catheters measure electrical activity and help define the exact location of the abnormal beat. They may also be used to stimulate the heart with tiny electrical impulses and to induce the arrhythmia for study and treatment.
6. The EP study may be followed immediately by radiofrequency ablation. An electrode catheter that has been threaded through the leg into the heart is placed at the site of the abnormal electrical pathway.
7. Radiofrequency energy is passed through the catheter.
8. The tip of the catheter heats up and "burns" the heart tissue where the abnormal pathway is located and destroys it.
9. The catheters are removed. Either firm pressure on the groin or a few stitches in the arm will close the site of the incision.

Duration: 2 to 6 hours.

What to expect when it's over:
It is necessary to lie flat for a few hours, the same as with angioplasty, to make sure there is no bleeding from the vessel where the catheter was introduced.

Patients usually go home the same day; in some cases they will be observed overnight in the hospital.

Recovery takes about 2 days and straining or lifting heavy objects should be avoided during that time.

In more than 90 percent of cases, abnormal heart rhythms are cured by ablation.

HEART VALVE REPLACEMENT AND REPAIR

There are four valves in the heart that allow blood to flow through the heart and prevent blood that's leaving it from coming back in. Any one of these valves may be diseased or damaged, but the most common valve operations involve the mitral and the aortic valves on the left side of the heart. The surgeon can repair or replace a diseased valve.

Part of the body operated on:
The heart and its valves.

Reasons for having the operation:
The valve can become so narrow that it does not allow enough blood to flow through it (stenotic).
The valve can leak, allowing a backflow of blood into chambers or vessels that it should be leaving (regurgitant).

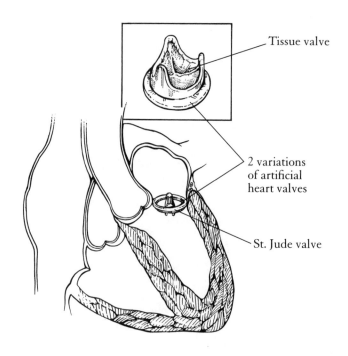

Tissue valve

2 variations of artificial heart valves

St. Jude valve

The malfunction of the valve is severe enough to cause symptoms of heart failure and/or chest pain, and may shorten life expectancy.

What could happen if you don't have the operation:
Increased pressure in the chambers of the heart and in the lungs, which could lead to worsening heart failure.

Factors that increase your risk of complications:
Diabetes.
Hypertension.
Obesity.
Peripheral vascular disease.
Previous stroke or heart attack.
Smoking.

Possible complications during and after surgery:
Excessive bleeding.
Heart attack.
Irregular heartbeat.
Stroke.
Wound infection.

Tests you may have to undergo:
Blood tests.
Cardiac catheterization (angiogram) for patients over fifty.
Chest X ray.
Echocardiogram (ultrasound imaging of the heart).
EKG.

Basic steps of the operation:
1. The surgery is done under general anesthesia.
2. An incision is made in the middle of the chest. The sternum (breastbone) is cut in half with a sternal saw.
3. The pericardium (fibrous outer covering of the heart) is opened and the heart is exposed.
4. The heart is connected by tubing to a heart-lung machine. The circulatory blood "bypasses" the heart; the pumping function

of the heart and the oxygenating of the lungs are taken over by the heart-lung machine.

5. Once connected to the heart-lung machine, the heart is stopped by the injection of a cold potassium solution.

6. Incisions are made to expose the valve, which is examined to determine the nature of the disease and extent of the problem. Depending on these findings, the valve is either repaired or replaced.

7. If the valve is replaced, the valve leaflets are excised and a new valve is sewn into place. Valves may be mechanical (made of metal alloys); biological (made from pig or cow tissue); or human (removed from a person who died).

8. After the valve is repaired or replaced, the heart is warmed, either naturally or by injecting a warm solution, and the incision exposing the valve is sewn closed.

9. Once the heart resumes its normal rhythm and function, the patient is disconnected from the heart-lung machine.

10. The sternum is closed with stainless-steel wire and the incisions in the chest are closed with absorbable sutures.

Duration: 4 to 5 hours.

What to expect when it's over:
Patients are brought to the intensive-care unit directly from the operating room.
Recovery occurs in stages:

Within the first 2 days, the breathing tube and chest tubes are removed and patients feel better.
Between the third and fourth day fatigue sets in; patients may actually feel worse, similar to having the flu.
Over the next week or so, patients begin to notice improved strength and appetite.

By the time patients are discharged, many normal activities such as walking up stairs, dining out, visiting friends, and sexual activity can be resumed. Strenuous activity will still cause fatigue.
Symptoms of valve disease like shortness of breath, chest pain, and lightheadedness generally disappear over time.

During the next 4 to 6 weeks, patients will notice continued improvement. Eating, sleeping, and bowel habits return to pre-operative patterns. Driving can be resumed around this time.

After 6 weeks, the levels of activity and stamina improve, especially if a patient does regular exercises, like walking.

Aches and pains from the incision may remain for about 2 to 3 months.

LUNG REMOVAL OR RESECTION

This surgery removes all or part of a lung.

Pneumonectomy (the entire lung).
Lobectomy (an entire lobe).
Wedge (small piece of lung).

Part of the body operated on:
The chest or thorax.

Reasons for having the operation:
Biopsy to determine whether a mass in the lungs is benign or malignant.
Removal of cancerous and benign tumors and surrounding areas.

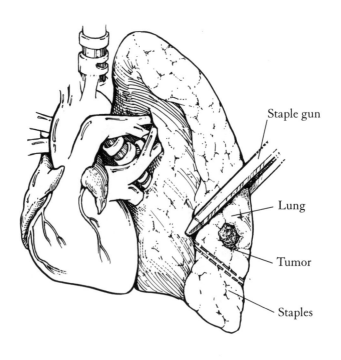

Staple gun

Lung

Tumor

Staples

What could happen if you don't have the operation:
Spread of cancer.
Death.

Factors that increase your risk of complications:
Diabetes.
Heart disease.
Kidney failure.
Liver disease.
Other types of lung disease.
Smoking.

Possible complications during and after surgery:
Bleeding.
Blood clots.
Heart attack.
Infection of tissues surrounding lungs.
Persistent air leakage from remaining lung.
Pneumonia.
Respiratory failure.
Stroke.

Tests you may have to undergo:
Biopsy.
Blood tests.
Bronchoscopy (see page 184).
Chest X rays.
CT scan.
EKG.
MRI.
Pulmonary function tests, to measure air passage through the lungs.

Basic steps of the operation:
1. General anesthesia is administered to the patient.
2. An incision is made in the chest between the ribs on the side of the chest, going under the armpit and around to the back.
3. The lung to be removed is deflated and examined. The veins, arteries, and airways leading to the lung, or to the lobe that is being removed, are divided.

4. All or part of the lung is removed.
5. A drainage tube is temporarily left in the chest.
6. The rib cage is repaired and the incisions are closed with sutures.

Duration: Pneumonectomy—2 hours. Lobectomy—3 hours. Wedge—2 hours.

What to expect when it's over:

Hospital stay of 3 to 7 days. Pain from the incision is controlled by medication.

Patients are taught breathing exercises to help strengthen the remaining lung.

Based on the location and the extent of the cancer, a treatment plan may include radiation therapy or chemotherapy.

Recovery takes about 4 to 6 weeks.

PACEMAKER INSERTION
OR REPLACEMENT

A pacemaker consists of a generator and leads (wires) that pace the rhythm of contraction and relaxation by sending out tiny electrical signals to the heart. It is placed in a person's body to keep the heart from beating too slowly.

Reasons for having the operation:
Pacemaker Insertion:
A malfunction in the body's system that conducts tiny electrical impulses in the heart; the natural pathway of electrical impulses is completely blocked; the heart's rhythm is very slow.
(In cases where the heartbeat is too fast, a different device called an ICD [implanted cardiovascular defibrillator] is implanted. This resembles a pacemaker but embodies a different set of functions.)

Pacemaker Replacement:
The battery of the pacemaker generator is depleted. Since the pacemaker is powered by a lithium-iodine battery, it will eventually

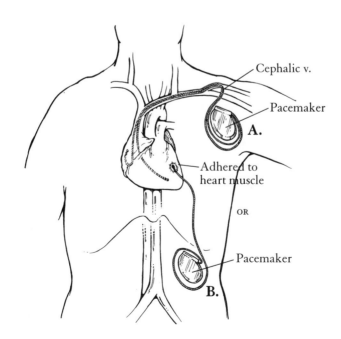

Cephalic v.

Pacemaker

A.

Adhered to heart muscle

OR

Pacemaker

B.

need to be replaced (in between 5 and 14 years). A signal is made by the pacemaker that tells the physician when the battery is nearing that time.

Changes in the patient's medical condition require revising the pacing system.

In rare cases, there are defects or a malfunction in the wires that go from the pacemaker to the heart, or there is an electronic defect or recall of the generator.

What could happen if you don't have the operation:
Dizziness, drowsiness, shortness of breath, or fainting.
A heartbeat that is too slow could lead to death.

Factors that increase your risk of complications:
Dementia.
Impaired ability of the blood to clot.
Very advanced heart disease or other critical illness.

Possible complications during and after surgery:
Arrhythmia (abnormal rhythm of the heart).
Failure of pacing system.
Infection.
Injury to the heart, lungs, blood vessels.

Tests you may have to undergo:
Blood tests.
Electrocardiogram (EKG).
Tests are also done to clarify whether a pacemaker is really needed and is likely to relieve symptoms. These include measuring and monitoring the electrical activity of the heart by various means:

Telemetry.
Holter monitoring (a continuous recording of an EKG while a patient goes about normal activities).
EP study (placing electrode catheters into the heart) (pages 191–93).

Basic steps of the operation:
The operation is done under local anesthesia with sedation. There are two types of insertions:

1. In one, a wire (lead) is inserted into a vein in the shoulder or upper chest. It is brought down to the heart.
2. The electrode at the end of the wire is attached inside the heart muscle that will receive the electrical impulse.
3. The other end of the wire is attached to the pacemaker (the pulse generator, made up of a battery and an electronic circuitry package), which is placed in a pocket between the skin and muscle of the upper chest, near the shoulder.
4. In the other method, an incision is made in the chest and the electrode is attached to the exterior surface of the heart. This requires general anesthesia.
5. The pacemaker is put into a pocket underneath the skin of the abdomen.

Duration: 1 to 2 hours.

If a pacemaker is being replaced, usually only the generator portion of the pacing system is removed. A new generator is inserted through an incision at the same location as the original one. Local anesthesia is used and the procedure takes about 30 to 40 minutes.

What to expect when it's over:
In most cases, patients can walk within an hour of surgery.
Discharge is the same day, unless the patient's original arrhythmic abnormality is potentially life-threatening.
There is minimal pain or stiffness at the site of the incisions.
Many patients resume activities the next day. Generally, patients are asked to wait 2 days before showering, 2 weeks for swimming, and 6 weeks for strenuous activities like tennis or basketball.
The pacemaker is not visible. Patients may be aware of the feeling of the pacemaker at first and they may have the urge to touch it until they have become accustomed to it.
Unusually strong sources of electrical interference such as microwaves, MRIs, and theft detectors could affect the pacemaker's operation. Patients need to learn which appliances or actions could cause interference and should be avoided.

14

Endocrine Surgery

PARATHYROIDECTOMY/ PARATHYROID SURGERY

Removal of one or more of the parathyroid glands, which are two pairs of small glands located near the thyroid. They produce a hormone that regulates the amount of calcium in the blood.

Part of the body operated on:
The neck.

Reasons for having the operation:
Benign tumor that is causing the glands to secrete excessive levels of hormones that control the amount of calcium in the blood (hyperparathyroidism). These tumors are rarely cancerous.

What could happen if you don't have the operation:
Hyperparathyroidism (or hypercalcemia—abnormally high levels of calcium in the blood) may lead to severe medical problems, including kidney failure and osteoporosis. If calcium levels should become very high, mental confusion, muscle weakness, and coma could occur.
The rare cancerous tumor would remain and possibly spread.

Factors that increase your risk of complications:
Underlying respiratory or cardiac problems.

Possible complications during and after surgery:
Hypoparathyroidism: When one or more of these glands is removed, the level of calcium in the body drops. This can cause uncomfortable spasms and tingling in the hands, lips, or feet. This is usually temporary until the remaining glands begin to function in place of the one that has been removed. Calcium pills, possibly with vitamin D, can be taken to correct this deficiency.

Tests you may have to undergo:
Blood tests.
Chest X ray.
EKG.
Radio nuclide scan (a nuclear scan to locate the parathyroid gland).

Basic steps of the operation:
1. Most patients have the surgery on an outpatient basis; anesthesia may be general or local.
2. An incision is made in the neck. The surgeon identifies the glands and notes the location of nearby nerves.
3. The gland or glands with tumors are removed.

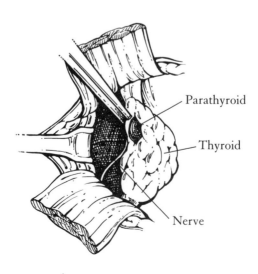

Parathyroid

Thyroid

Nerve

4. About 10 to 30 percent of patients have thyroid abnormalities found at the time of parathyroid surgery that may require partial or total removal of the thyroid. These can be removed at the same time using the same incision and anesthesia.
5. The skin is sutured to close it.

Duration: 45 minutes.

What to expect when it's over:

After the sutures are removed, the area is sprayed with collodion, a clear plastic covering that comes off on its own after a few days.

Numbing medication lasts about 12 hours; thereafter pain is controlled by oral medication. Most patients can eat and drink normally, but there may be pain on swallowing for 12 to 24 hours.

Patients can shower, but should not submerge the wound for 7 days.

There will be a scar, which can be minimized through smaller incision size, placement of the incision, and plastic surgery. Generally, the scar is not noticeable after 6 months except in individuals with wound-healing problems. Sunburn can damage new skin and cause the scar to be more noticeable. Exposure to sun should be avoided.

After local anesthesia, most patients can return to work within a few days of surgery; after general anesthesia, the return to normal activities is slightly longer—5 to 7 days.

THYROIDECTOMY/THYROID SURGERY

Removal of all or part of the thyroid gland. This gland secretes the hormone thyroxin that plays an important part in the body's metabolism.

Part of the body operated on:
The neck.

Reasons for having the operation:
To remove a cancerous tumor.
Malfunction of the gland, which results in abnormal levels of hormones in the bloodstream.
To remove a goiter, a benign growth that may cause difficulty in swallowing and/or breathing.

What could happen if you don't have the operation:
Spread of cancer.

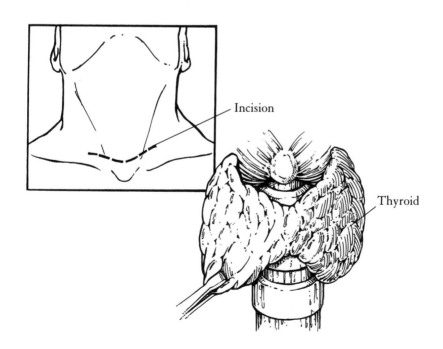

Incision

Thyroid

Continued production of abnormal levels of hormone secretion, leading to hyperthyroidism or hypothyroidism.

Symptoms of goiter could continue and lead to blockage of breathing, requiring emergency tracheostomy.

Factors that increase your risk of complications:
Underlying respiratory or cardiac problems.

Possible complications during and after surgery:
The nerves that control the voice are temporarily affected by the removal of the thyroid, which could cause difficulties with voice projection and making high-pitched sounds for up to a few months. Permanent change is rare.

In about 8 percent of patients who have thyroid surgery, the parathyroid glands do not function properly immediately after the surgery. This is usually temporary and causes the blood calcium level to drop below normal (hypocalcemia) leading to numbness and tingling in the hands, soles of the feet, and lips; other symptoms include a crawling sensation in the skin, muscle cramps, or severe headache. Calcium supplements are given to treat the condition and it usually disappears in 7 to 10 days.

Tests you may have to undergo:
Blood tests.
Chest X ray.
EKG.

Basic steps of the operation:
1. This is usually done as outpatient surgery, with general or local anesthesia.
2. An incision is made along a natural crease in the neck. The parathyroid glands and the nerves are identified; the thyroid gland is exposed.
3. The abnormal thyroid is removed and sent for laboratory analysis.
4. The incision is sutured and the skin is sewn together.
Duration: 1 hour.

What to expect when it's over:
After the sutures are removed, the area is sprayed with collodion, a clear plastic covering that comes off on its own after a few days. Patients can bathe but should not submerge the incision for 7 days. A moisturizer applied to the wound improves healing.

Numbing medication lasts about 8 hours; thereafter, there is likely to be pain on swallowing, which can be controlled by oral medication.

If local anesthesia is used, patients are back to normal activity within 2 to 3 days; recovery time may be longer—3 to 4 days—with general anesthesia.

There will be a scar, but techniques that include smaller incision size, placement of the incision, and use of hypoallergenic suture material minimize scarring. Since the skin is closed using a plastic surgery technique, the scar is not noticeable after 6 months except in the rare patient with wound-healing problems. Sunburn can damage new skin and cause the scar to be more noticeable. Exposure to sun should be avoided.

Patients who have undergone local anesthesia will likely be able to return to work in a few days; it will be longer after general anesthesia—perhaps one or two weeks after surgery. Patients are encouraged to move their heads normally. As soon as patients have full head and neck mobility, driving can be safely resumed. For most patients, this takes from 1 to 3 days.

It may be necessary to take hormone supplements on a permanent basis, prescribed by your physician.

For thyroid cancers, there may be follow-up treatment, including therapy with radioactive iodine.

15

Gastrointestinal Surgery

COLECTOMY/COLORECTAL RESECTION

Removal of all or part of the large intestine (the colon), possibly including the rectum.

Part of the body operated on:
The intestine, abdomen, and/or the pelvic region.

Reasons for having the operation:
Cancer (tumor/malignancy).
Inflammation, bleeding, blockage, or rupture of the intestine.
Diverticulitis (inflammation involving small sacs protruding from the lining of the intestine).

What could happen if you don't have the operation:
Spread of cancer.
Pain and swelling in the abdomen.
An obstructed intestine and inability to pass stools; complete blockage can be fatal.
Life-threatening infection or bleeding.

Factors that increase your risk of complications:
Bleeding disorders.

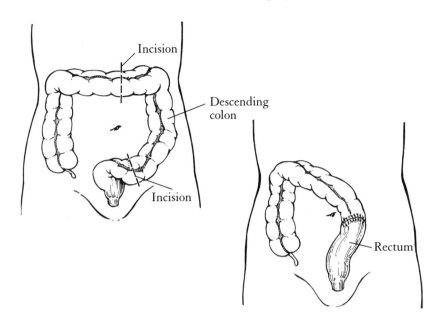

Heart or lung diseases.
Steroid dependency.

Possible complications during and after surgery:
Anastomotic leak (the connection between the two ends of the
  bowel may not seal and stool could leak through).
Bleeding.
Blood clots in leg veins.
Infection.
Pneumonia.
Recurrence of cancer.

Tests you may have to undergo:
Blood tests.
Chest X ray.
Colonoscopy (an examination inside the colon by means of a long,
  flexible tube).
CT scan (abdomen and pelvis; possibly the chest).
EKG.
Possibly ultrasound and barium X-ray studies (ingestion of a chemi-
  cal that enables X rays to detect abnormalities in the colon).

Basic steps of the operation:
1. General anesthesia is administered to the patient.
2. The surgeon makes an incision into the abdomen.
3. The diseased part of the colon is separated and removed.
4. The ends of the bowel are rejoined.
5. The abdomen is sutured and closed.

Duration: 4 hours.

If the cancerous section of bowel that was removed was so low down in the rectum or anus that not enough healthy bowel remains for anastomosis, the patient will need a colostomy. This is an operation in which the colon is attached to the abdomen by creating an opening (stoma) in order to deposit feces into a colostomy pouch.

In some cases, it isn't immediately clear that the seal between the loops of the bowel that were rejoined is strong enough. An upstream temporary colostomy or ileostomy (if small bowel is used) is then performed and left in place while the downstream bowel is healing. The colostomy is reversed in about 6 to 8 weeks when it's clear that the seal is holding well.

When a section of the small intestine is brought to the surgically created opening, the surgery is called an ileostomy.

What to expect when it's over:

There is usually pain from the incision; most patients receive intravenous pain medication after surgery through a patient-controlled pump.

Patients may also have gas pains before they start to regain bowel function.

A liquid diet is resumed once there is no danger of the patient vomiting. Most surgeons will then increase the diet in line with the patient's ability to tolerate additional items, and the recovery of bowel function as judged by the passage of flatus or stool.

Patients remain in the hospital for about 1 week.

Those who have a colostomy pouch are taught before they leave the hospital how to take care of the opening and the skin around it and how to use the pouch.

GASTRIC BYPASS

*By creating a mechanism to bypass 95 percent of the stomach,
this operation results in a substantial decrease in the amount
of food that a person eats.*

Part of the body operated on:
The stomach and the small intestine, through the upper abdomen.

Reasons for having the operation:
Morbid obesity (at least 100 pounds over ideal weight).
Obesity-related medical problems (diabetes, hypertension, sleep apnea) and a weight that is about 100 pounds over the ideal.
Having either of these conditions and a failure to lose weight through a combined regimen of diet and exercise.
Reversal of obesity, which, after smoking, is the second most common contributor to factors leading to death.

What could happen if you don't have the operation:
If a patient is not able to lose substantial amounts of weight by other means like diet and exercise, he would remain obese. Many major medical problems are caused by obesity, like type II diabetes. Others

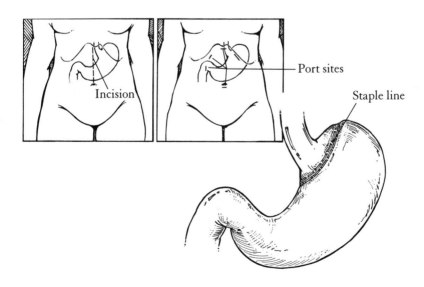

Incision

Port sites

Staple line

are aggravated by it, including: hypertension; joint problems like osteoarthritis; respiratory problems; cardiovascular disease; congestive heart failure; varicose veins; increased risk of breast and uterine cancer; gastroesophageal reflux disease; urinary incontinence; and some types of headache.

Factors that increase your risk of complications:
Extreme or morbid obesity.
Other serious medical problems, including: pulmonary diseases, cardiac disease.
Smoking.
Steroid medication.
Many of the same factors that increase the risk of surgery—obesity, disease—are also improved by the surgery. Patients should do a risk/benefit analysis on an individual basis with their doctor and determine whether there is more to gain by taking on the risk of surgery than there is by continuing to be obese.

Possible complications during and after surgery:
Blood clot or embolus (clump of material in the bloodstream that leads to an obstruction of a lung artery).
Incisional hernia (a bulge in the abdominal wall).
Infection in the wound.
Leakage of intestinal contents.

Tests you may have to undergo:
Blood tests.
Chest X ray.
Echocardiogram (ultrasound study that looks at structure of the heart).
EKG.
Tests to determine medical problems like sleep apnea (breathing stops during sleep) or other breathing problems.

Basic steps of the operation:
1. Surgery is done either by laparoscopic surgery or open surgery. Both types are done with general anesthesia.
2. *Open surgery:* An upper abdominal incision is made from the bottom of the breastbone to the belly button. *Laparoscopic*

surgery: 5 small incisions are made, 4 of which are about the width of a finger. One is under the breastbone, another under the belly button, and two in the right upper abdomen. The fifth incision, in the left upper abdomen, is larger, about three finger-widths, and enables a stapling device to enter the body.

3. The top of the stomach is divided in two by the stapling device. This area is separated or partitioned from the rest of the stomach to create a small pouch, of an ounce or less, at the bottom of the esophagus where it enters the stomach. The pouch stretches in time and the size of the pouch is very important. If it's too small, the patient can't eat; if it's too large, the patient doesn't lose enough weight.

4. The upper portion of the small intestine is cut and then re-attached in a different configuration. Instead of a single line, it is transformed into a Y-shaped tube. One arm of the Y connects the section of the small intestine that comes out of the stomach (the duodenum) to the rest of the intestinal tube, at a new point lower down. This brings the gastric juices out of the stomach into the intestine. The other arm of the Y is attached higher up to the newly created small pouch (this area is called the stoma). This brings the food that the patient has eaten into the intestine. Attachments are done by sutures or staples.

5. The food and the gastric juices come through the two separate tubes and meet in a new location in the small intestine, where digestion now begins.

6. The incisions in the muscles and the skin are closed.

Duration: 3 to 4 hours.

What to expect when it's over:
In both kinds of surgery, patients stay about 3 to 4 days in the hospital. With open surgery, it takes about 4 to 6 weeks to return to normal activities. If done laparoscopically, recovery is about 2 to 3 weeks.

In the first day or two, patients have a patient-controlled analgesia (PCA) pump for pain. By the time patients leave the hospital, they are on oral medication for pain, like Tylenol with codeine, and will continue taking it for about another week.

Patients are limited to pureed food for 4 to 6 weeks after surgery, and then slowly progress to normal foods.

Thereafter, patients' eating habits change drastically:

> They can't eat the quantity of food they did before the operation. Food enters the small pouch, empties slowly, and causes a person to feel full very quickly.
>
> Overeating can be very uncomfortable and may result in vomiting.
>
> Eating sweets may cause nausea, lightheadedness, and extreme tiredness.
>
> Eating too much fat can result in diarrhea and cramps.

Weight loss varies widely depending on factors that include a patient's age, starting weight, commitment to exercise, and a diet that avoids sweets, junk food, and fried foods. Initially, heavier patients tend to lose more pounds, but lighter patients are more likely to come close to their ideal weight. Eighty-five percent of patients lose two-thirds of their excess weight; 95 percent lose at least one half.

HEMORRHOIDECTOMY/
HEMORRHOID REMOVAL

Hemorrhoids are enlarged and swollen veins extending out from the lining of the anal area. They are often caused by excessive strain when moving feces. Hemorrhoids can be removed surgically when symptoms are too difficult to manage and other treatment options fail.

Part of the body operated on:
The rectal area.

Reasons for having the operation:
Rectal bleeding.
Pain when defecating.
Hemorrhoids that have slipped down and out of position (prolapsed) can lead to mucous discharge and itching.

What could happen if you don't have the operation:
Treatment by other methods—including change in diet and bowel habits, sitz baths, use of topical creams, medication, or injection of

Rectum

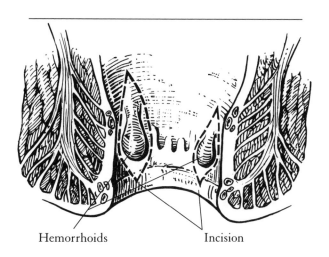

Hemorrhoids   Incision

a chemical by a doctor to destroy the hemorrhoids—may resolve the problem, especially if the hemorrhoids are small. The hemorrhoid may respond to banding: a tight band is placed by a specially designed instrument on the neck of the hemorrhoid, which eventually withers and falls off. If other treatments fail, symptoms could continue and become very uncomfortable.
In rare cases, bleeding could lead to anemia.
Prolapsed hemorrhoids could lead to a clot in the vein and more intense pain.

Factors that increase your risk of complications:
Other serious medical conditions.

Possible complications during and after surgery:
Bleeding.
Infection.
Mild fecal incontinence (rare).
Urinary retention, especially in patients older than forty.

Tests you may have to undergo:
Blood tests.
Chest X ray.
EKG.
Proctoscopy (examination of the rectal area through a viewing tube).
Sigmoidoscopy (examination of the rectum and the last part of the colon through a viewing tube).

Basic steps of the operation:
1. The operation is performed under general or spinal anesthesia.
2. An instrument is inserted in the rectum to pull out and expose the hemorrhoid.
3. The tissue to be removed is clamped and cut off.
4. The remaining edges are sewn closed.
Duration: 1 hour.

What to expect when it's over:
There may be significant pain for 2 to 3 days, which is controlled by oral pain medication.

Some spasm of the rectum may occur. Sitting in warm baths helps discomfort.

Stool is likely to be liquid at first, then more formed bowel movements will resume. It is important not to become constipated, and stool softeners taken by mouth are often required for several months.

Soiling may occur for 1 to 2 weeks, while sphincter muscles, cut during surgery, regain their normal function.

Diet will be restricted to soft foods for the first couple of days after surgery.

LAPAROSCOPIC CHOLECYSTECTOMY / GALLBLADDER REMOVAL

Removal of the gallbladder, a small organ under the liver that stores bile for digestion. When it's removed, its function is taken over by the liver.

In laparoscopic surgery, small incisions are made in the abdomen for visibility through an endoscope and to insert instruments. Open surgery uses a large incision with direct vision and is infrequently done now.

Part of the body operated on:
The gallbladder, through the upper abdomen.

Reasons for having the operation:
Gallstones (solidified chemicals in the gallbladder) which are causing blockages, pain, or infection.

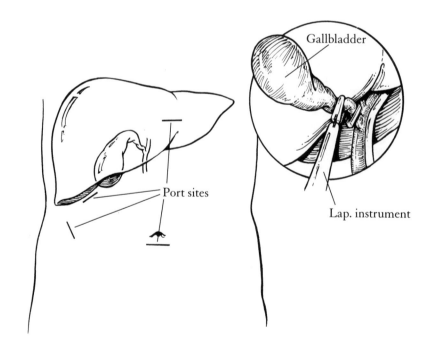

Gallbladder

Port sites

Lap. instrument

What could happen if you don't have the operation:
Continued attacks of pain.
Migration of gallstones, leading to life-threatening inflammation of the pancreas (pancreatitis) or obstruction of the bile duct, which causes jaundice (yellowing of the skin).

Factors that increase your risk of complications:
Heart or lung disease.

Possible complications during and after surgery:
Bleeding.
Damage to the bile duct.
Damage to the intestine.
Infection.
Leakage of bile into the abdomen.
Leg vein blood clots.

Tests you may have to undergo:
Blood tests.
Chest X ray.
EKG.
Ultrasound scanning of the abdomen (sonography).

Basic steps of the operation:
1. The patient is anesthetized.
2. The skin is cleansed and 4 small (1 centimeter or less) incisions are made.
3. Gas is inserted into the abdominal cavity to make the gallbladder easier to see. A laparoscope is placed through one of the incisions to project an image of the area to be operated on.
4. Instruments are inserted through the other incisions to grasp the gallbladder and to free it from its attachments to vessels and ducts. (In rare cases, based on the examination of the gallbladder once it is visible, the surgeon may conclude that its condition requires removal by means of open surgery. The operation will then be switched to one in which a large incision is made.)
5. The gallbladder is removed through one of the incisions.

6. If gallstones are found in the bile duct, those stones may also be removed during the procedure, or removed later via an endoscope.
7. The incisions are closed with sutures.

Duration: 1½ hours.

What to expect when it's over:

Mild nausea. Mild pain at the site of the incisions.

Hospital stay of 12 to 24 hours.

Patient is able to eat and function normally within the first few weeks after the operation.

It takes 2 to 4 weeks to have full return of stamina.

LAPAROSCOPIC FUNDOPLICATION/ ESOPHAGEAL SURGERY/ ANTIREFLUX SURGERY

An operation to treat gastroesophageal reflux disease (GERD), which is the regurgitation of acidic juices from the stomach into the esophagus. Reflux is usually caused by a defect in the muscle that connects the esophagus with the stomach.

Part of the body operated on:
The lower esophagus and the upper stomach, reached through the abdomen.

Reasons for having the operation:
Reflux is so severe that it requires long-term medication, or the patient does not respond well to medication.

What could happen if you don't have the operation:
Patient would need to take medication for the rest of his life.
Reflux often causes inflammation and damage to the esophagus and occasionally to the lungs and vocal cords.

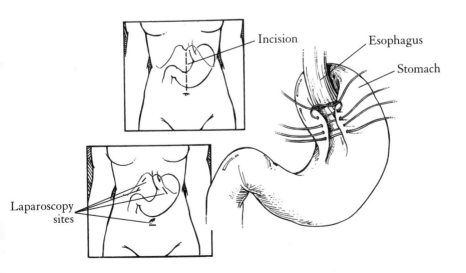

Incision   Esophagus

Stomach

Laparoscopy sites

Risk of developing esophageal cancer is increased.
Symptoms of heartburn and regurgitation will continue.

Factors that increase your risk of complications:
Lung and heart disease.

Possible complications during and after surgery:
Bloating, flatulence.
Perforation of the stomach or esophagus (in about 1 percent of patients).
Reoperation because of bleeding or perforations.
Swallowing problems.

Tests you may have to undergo:
Any one or all of the following tests may be required:

Manometry: passing a small flexible tube through the nose into the esophagus and stomach in order to measure pressure and function of the esophagus.
pH probe: measures the amount of acid refluxed into the esophagus over 24 hours.
Upper endoscopy: a flexible tube with a visualization device goes into the mouth and down through the stomach. It enables the surgeon to obtain small tissue samples, which can be studied to confirm esophageal inflammation and exclude other diseases.
Upper GI series or barium swallow X ray: shows acid reflux and inflammation of the esophagus. It also shows whether the patient has a hiatal hernia, a condition in which the upper part of the stomach has moved up into the chest through a small opening in the diaphragm.

Basic steps of the operation:
1. The patient is administered general anesthesia.
2. Fundoplication surgery can be done either by traditional methods in which the abdomen is opened with an incision of about 8 inches, or through laparoscopy, in which 4 to 5 incisions of a half inch each are made in the abdomen. Most cases are now repaired through laparoscopy.

3. The top of the stomach is loosely wrapped around the bottom of the esophagus to create a valve.
4. The surgeon raises the liver to expose the junction between the stomach and the esophagus.
5. A space is created behind the esophagus and the fundus (top) of the stomach. The stomach is freed from its attachments. The fundus is then pulled behind the esophagus and secured in place.
6. For more severe cases of reflux, the top of the stomach is completely wrapped around the esophagus and is sewn to the esophagus. In less severe cases, the wrap goes only part of the way around and is also sewn to the esophagus. A partial wrap causes less gas bloat and less difficulty in swallowing, but a complete wrap controls reflux more effectively. Patients with abnormal function of the esophagus may tolerate a complete wrap less well.
7. Laparoscopy leads to a quicker recovery and fewer complications, but it may not be appropriate for patients who have had previous abdominal surgery or other preexisting medical conditions. In rare cases (about 5 percent), the surgeon has to switch from laparoscopy to traditional open surgery during the procedure.
8. The incisions in both types of surgery are closed with stitches or surgical tape and covered with bandages.

Duration: 4 hours.

What to expect when it's over:
More than 90 percent of patients have no further reflux after surgery.

Upon waking, patients often have a tube leading from their nose into their stomach to decompress the area around the wrap.

Diet is restricted. Only liquids are allowed the first day after the tube is removed and solely soft foods for several weeks thereafter.

After laparoscopy, patients usually leave the hospital in 1 to 2 days; after open surgery, the hospital stay is 4 to 7 days. For about 2 weeks after surgery, patients take acid-reducing medication.

It takes about 1 to 2 weeks to return to full activity after laparoscopy; 4 to 6 weeks after open surgery.

A follow-up appointment should be scheduled for 7 to 10 days after discharge.

The new valve mechanism may cause resistance to the passage of food, causing more air to be swallowed. Patients often experience periods of bloating from gas. For 2 to 3 hours after eating, the wrap makes the increased air difficult to belch. Patients may also have abdominal distention, nausea, and an increase in flatulence. These usually resolve over time.

Patients may also have difficulty swallowing for about 6 weeks because of swelling at the site. If this doesn't go away, the area may be treated by stretching it with a balloon. In rare cases, a patient may need another operation to treat swallowing difficulty.

A soft diet eases most post-surgical difficulties.

PANCREATECTOMY/PANCREAS SURGERY

Removal of part of the pancreas, an organ that lies behind the stomach and connects to the small intestine (the duodenum) by a duct. The main function of the pancreas is to secrete digestive enzymes into the intestines and to secrete hormones, including insulin, that regulate blood sugar levels.

Part of the body operated on:
The pancreas, through the upper abdomen.

Reasons for having the operation:
Cancer, which is often difficult to detect. Its symptoms, which include pain, nausea, vomiting, and jaundice, may not appear until more advanced stages of the disease.

Infrequently, if medication does not work, very severe pain from chronic pancreatitis (inflammation of the pancreas) may be treated with surgery.

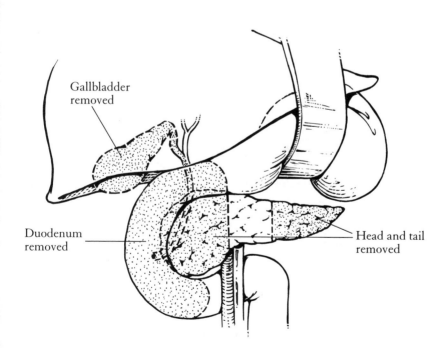

Gallbladder removed

Duodenum removed

Head and tail removed

What could happen if you don't have the operation:
The cancer could spread and cause death.
Pain of pancreatitis would continue.

Factors that increase your risk of complications:
Other serious medical problems, such as diabetes, or heart or lung disease.

Possible complications during and after surgery:
Blood clots in leg veins.
Diabetes.
Infection.
Malabsorption (impaired absorption of nutrients due to lack of pancreatic enzymes).

Tests you may have to undergo:
Blood tests.
CT scan.
EKG.
ERCP (Endosopic Retrograde Cholangio Pancreatography): a flexible, lighted viewing tube is passed down the throat to the upper part of the small intestine; a dye is inserted and X rays are taken.

Basic steps of the operation:
1. General anesthesia is administered.
2. An incision is made in the abdomen.
3. Other organs, especially the liver, are checked for spread of cancer that may not have been detected in pre-surgical testing. If cancer has spread, the pancreas may not be removed and treatment will be done with chemotherapy instead. If the cancer is localized in the pancreas, the operation will proceed with removal of the diseased sections.
4. The gallbladder is then removed if it is involved with the disease process.
5. Depending on the location of the cancer, a portion of the pancreas, such as its tail or head end, may be removed. In other cases, the head of the pancreas and the section of the stomach where it meets the small intestine may have to be removed.

6. A gastrostomy tube may be inserted in the stomach to allow a comfortable recovery. This may remain for about 10 days.
7. Ducts and intestines that have been cut during surgery are re-connected.
8. The incision is stapled closed.

Duration: 4 hours.

What to expect when it's over:

Hospital stay is usually 5 to 12 days.

Pain is controlled through medication. Patient can use PCA (patient-controlled analgesia) to control pain.

After the bowel is able to function, patients will be given clear liquid. Diet will be restricted to low-fat food for about 6 to 8 weeks.

Patients often need additional chemotherapy or radiation to treat the cancer.

In some cases, patients may need to take medication to supply insulin or enzymes for digestion.

Long-term recovery of gastrointestinal function is excellent.

PEPTIC ULCER SURGERY

This operation alters the stomach anatomy to reduce the amount of acid produced in the digestive process. When too much peptic acid is produced, it begins to eat away at the tissues lining the intestinal tract, usually the lower stomach and upper small intestine (duodenum). A peptic ulcer is the raw, painful area that results. By cutting certain nerves that send the message to the stomach to produce the acid, the operation reduces the amount of acid and enables the ulcer to heal.

Part of the body operated on:
The abdomen.

Reasons for having the operation:
Desire to avoid lifelong medication.
Failure of medication to reduce acid and to heal the ulcers.
Relief from pain, appetite changes, nausea, and bloating.

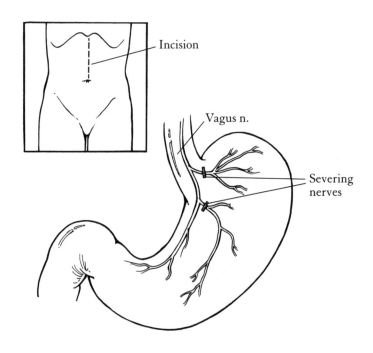

Incision

Vagus n.

Severing nerves

What could happen if you don't have the operation:
Bleeding from the ulcer.
Leakage of digestive juices to the pancreas.
Need to stay on medications.
Obstruction in the passage from the stomach to the duodenum.
Perforation of the stomach or duodenum.
Peritonitis (inflammation of the lining of the abdominal cavity).
Recurrent attacks of pain.

Factors that increase your risk of complications:
Obesity.
Severe cardiac or pulmonary disease.

Possible complications during and after surgery:
Bleeding.
Blood clots in leg veins.
Diarrhea and cramps at meals.
Infection.
Pneumonia.

Tests you may have to undergo:
Blood tests.
EKG.
Upper endoscopy.
Upper gastrointestinal series: X ray, study of upper GI tract with barium or dye.
X ray.

Basic steps of the operation:
1. The patient has general anesthesia. A catheter is placed into the bladder and a tube is placed in the stomach via the nose. An incision is made in the upper abdomen.
2. The surgeon examines the stomach area, identifies the many small branches of the vagus nerves, and severs them from the stomach.
Duration: 1 hour.
3. In some cases, it may be necessary to remove a portion of the

stomach and reconnect it to the small intestine. Drains may be left in.

Duration: 2 hours.

4. The abdominal incision is closed with sutures.

What to expect when it's over:

Tubes are left in the stomach and bladder for 3 days. Pain from the incision lasts about 1 week. Medication is initially patient-controlled analgesia, then oral medication.

In the first 3 to 5 days after surgery, food intake is limited to clear liquids and soft foods.

16

General Surgery

APPENDECTOMY

Removal of an infected and inflamed appendix (a small tube a little more than 3 inches long, jutting out from the area where the large intestine and small intestine meet; it has no known function). Appendicitis usually comes on very quickly and is indicated by severe pain in the lower right side of the abdomen. Surgery is generally done on an emergency basis.

Part of the body operated on:
The appendix, through the lower abdomen.

Reasons for having the operation:
To relieve pain, fever, and nausea.
To prevent the spread of infection.

What could happen if you don't have the operation:
The appendix may rupture, causing peritonitis, which is a serious infection of the abdominal cavity; death is likely if untreated.

Factors that increase your risk of complications:
Heart disease.
Malignancy.

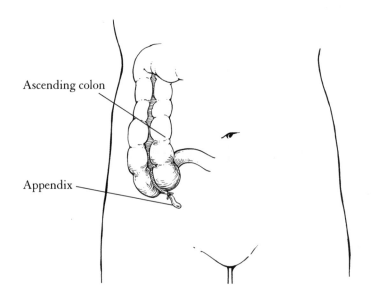

Ascending colon

Appendix

Obesity.
Pulmonary disease.

Possible complications during and after surgery:
Bleeding.
Delayed return of bowel function.
Hernia.
Intraabdominal abscess.
Pneumonia.
Wound infection.

Tests you may have to undergo:
Abdominal X ray.
Blood tests: blood count and clotting.
Chest X ray.
Pregnancy test. (A pregnant patient would need to have a different
   anesthesia and a monitor for the fetal heart rate.)
Urinalysis.

Basic steps of the operation:
   1. The patient is administered general anesthesia.
   2. The surgeon makes an incision in the lower right abdomen.

3. The inflamed appendix is freed from adjacent organs (small intestine, right ovary in females, abdominal wall) by blunt finger dissection. (A finger instead of an instrument is used to do the dissection.)

4. The base of the appendix, which is attached to the large intestine at the cecum (the pouch where the large intestine begins), is clamped and severed. The appendix is removed from the abdomen.

5. The stump that remains from the appendix is tied off, "dunked" into the wall of the cecum, and sewn closed to minimize the risk of leakage or adhesions.

6. The abdomen is irrigated and the incisions are closed with tiny staples or sutures.

Duration: 1 hour.

What to expect when it's over:

The patient can walk within several hours of the operation. Hospitalization lasts from 1 to 3 days.

Return to most normal activities occurs within 2 to 3 weeks; resumption of activities like weightlifting or jogging may take a few weeks longer.

CATARACT REMOVAL

The lens inside the eye turns cloudy so that light passing through the eye is seen as a blur. This cloudy lens, or cataract, is removed and is replaced with a synthetic lens.

Part of the body operated on:
The eye.

Reasons for having the operation:
Blurred vision, glare, or halo around lights that cannot be improved with a change in eyeglasses.
In some cases, although a patient can live with blurred vision, the cataract is so dense that surgery is recommended to prevent complications in the future.
Lens-induced glaucoma or elevation of pressure in the eye (very rare).

What could happen if you don't have the operation:
The cataract may harden and make surgery more difficult and complicated.

Factors that increase your risk of complications:
Corneal weakness.
Small pupils.
Unstable general medical health.
Various forms of glaucoma.

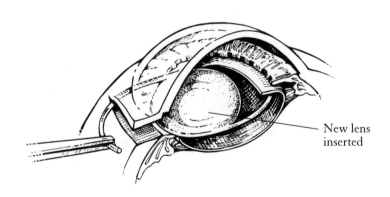

New lens inserted

Possible complications during and after surgery:
Bad positioning of the new lens.
Bleeding (minor or major hemorrhage).
Complications (in a fraction of a percent of those operated on) could lead to blindness.
Infection.

Tests you may have to undergo:
A scan (ultrasound test) to decide the strength of the new lens.
Blood tests.
Chest X ray.
EKG.
Other eye tests, such as specular microscopy, may be ordered by the ophthalmologist if there appears to be a weakness of the cornea.

Basic steps of the operation:
1. The eye is anesthetized with topical and intraocular anesthesia. This causes fewer complications than the older method of injection of an anesthetic behind the eyeball.
2. A small incision is made into the cornea. An opening is made in the front surface of the lens.
3. In a process called phacoemulsification, the cloudy lens is broken up into small pieces, or liquefied, ultrasonically. It is then suctioned out. The sac of the original lens is left intact.
4. In older methods of cataract removal, which are sometimes still used today, a slightly larger incision is made and the lens is taken out as a whole by means of a surgical tool.
5. In both cases, the back part of the lens is left to support the replacement lens.
6. A plastic lens is then folded like a taco, passed through the incision, and placed inside the sac. It is attached with flexible tabs held in place by the eye sac.
7. The incision is closed with stromal hydration, which is sterile salt water. In rare cases, it is closed with sutures.
Duration: 30 minutes for one eye.

What to expect when it's over:
The patient leaves the hospital the same day.

It may be necessary to wear a patch and an eye shield for a short time; sunglasses are recommended. The eye may be red and sensitive and there may be swelling of the area. Eyedrops usually relieve uncomfortable symptoms.

It is important not to bend or lift until the eye is healed, primarily if the incision is large.

Recovery is generally within 2 days, especially with small-incision surgery.

The success rate of the surgery is about 90 to 98 percent. Vision will be improved, although in some cases the presence of other eye diseases may limit the improvement. For most, it is likely that a new eyeglass prescription will be necessary.

If the sac behind the new lens becomes cloudy in a few months or years, laser treatment can be done on the sac to sharpen the vision again.

CEREBRAL ANEURYSM REPAIR

This operation seals off an aneurysm in a blood vessel in the brain. An aneurysm is a ballooning in an artery, caused by the pressure of blood flowing through a weakened area. Surgery is done to prevent the aneurysm from leaking or rupturing.

Part of the body operated on:
The head, behind the hairline.

Reasons for having the operation:
To prevent stroke and/or death due to rupture. To relieve symptoms, which include severe headache, double vision, and nausea. The risk of surgery in patients under the age of 70 is almost always less than the risk of catastrophic rupture without surgery.

What could happen if you don't have the operation:
The aneurysm could rupture, causing a stroke or death.

Factors that increase your risk of complications:
Advanced age.
Poor neurological condition (previous stroke, bleeding and stroke).

Possible complications during and after surgery:
Hemorrhage.
Stroke.

Tests you may have to undergo:
Blood tests.
Cerebral angiogram.
Chest X ray.
CT Scan.
EKG.
MRI.

Basic steps of the operation:
1. The patient is administered general anesthesia.
2. An incision is made behind the hairline.

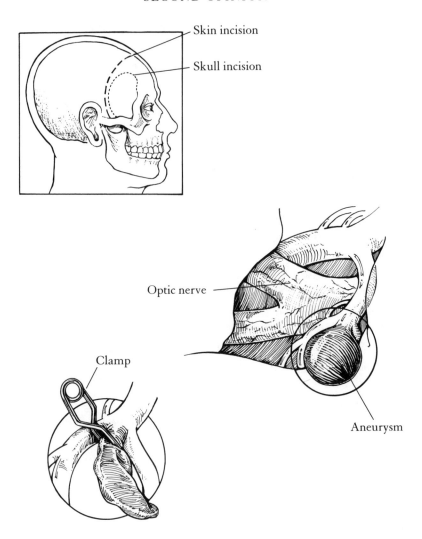

Skin incision

Skull incision

Optic nerve

Clamp

Aneurysm

3. A tiny saw opens a "trap door" in the skull.
4. A clip is placed on the aneurysm during microsurgery. The clip squeezes the aneurysm; the artery remains open and the blood flows normally to the brain.
5. The bone is screwed back into place at the end of surgery and the incision is closed.

Duration: 5 hours.

What to expect when it's over:
Usually 2 days in the hospital. Minor headache, which can last several weeks, is generally controlled with oral pain medication.
Resumption of normal activities takes about 1 month, return to full-time work about 4 to 8 weeks.

CLEFT LIP REPAIR

Creating a single, aligned upper lip, usually during the first three months of life, for a child who is born with a lip that has an abnormal split. If the condition is not treated in infancy, the operation can also be performed on older children or adults.

Part of the body operated on:
Upper lip; possibly the nose.
In some cases, patients who have a cleft lip also have a cleft palate, which is a gap in the roof of the mouth. It causes problems with hearing, speech, and eating and is repaired in a separate operation.

Reasons for having the operation:
To join together lip segments so that the face is normal in appearance and the lips function properly. The operation repairs any size split, including a little notch, a separation that goes halfway up the lip, or a complete division that goes into the nose.
To repair a nasal deformity that often accompanies a cleft lip, in which the tip of the nose is pushed down and out on the side of the cleft and flattened, and the nasal septum is bent.

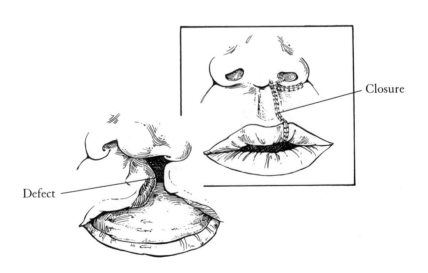

Closure

Defect

What could happen if you don't have the operation:
The patient will have an obvious facial deformity, an inability to pucker the lips or make whistling sounds, and may have difficulty in creating the lip seal that is necessary to nurse.
Speech problems do not usually occur in children who have a cleft lip alone, but they may be present if there is also a cleft palate.

Factors that increase your risk of complications:
Heart or lung problems.
Premature birth.
Very small size at birth.

Possible complications during and after surgery:
Bleeding.
Infection.
Unsightly scarring.
Wound (lip) separation.

Tests you may have to undergo:
In a healthy child, no basic tests are needed.
If the child is unhealthy, the extent of testing depends on the degree of illness.

Basic steps of the operation:
The operation may be performed as early as 1 month after birth. If the child has health problems, the operation is more likely to be done when the child is at least 3 months old.

1. General anesthesia is used to keep a very young child still.
2. The surgeon uses a knife to separate the lip segments from the underlying bone.
3. Once the lips are released, the segments are pulled together, lined up, and put into proper position and contour. They are sewn in place with very fine sutures. Layered closure is used to minimize scarring.
4. Correction of associated nasal deformities is done by freeing cartilage from its abnormal positions and reshaping it so that it does not appear flattened. The work is done from inside the nose so that incisions are not visible on the surface of the nose.

Duration: 1½ hours.

What to expect when it's over:

Regular child-strength Tylenol is generally given for pain.

Patients can breastfeed immediately after surgery; recovery takes about 1 day.

Surgery usually produces a very normal-appearing lip. In cases where a patient forms abnormal scar tissue, a brief outpatient procedure may be necessary to correct it.

HERNIA REPAIR

This is an operation to repair an abdominal wall defect or rupture. The hernia is made up of a sac of the abdominal lining (peritoneum) filled with abdominal organs, usually in the area of the groin. The weak area of abdominal wall where the bulge occurred is strengthened through surgery.

Part of the body operated on:
The abdomen and the groin.

Reasons for having the operation:
To remove an uncomfortable and unsightly bulge; less commonly, to treat an intestinal obstruction.

What could happen if you don't have the operation:
The protruding bulge would slowly enlarge and pain would increase. This could lead to serious complications resulting in a disruption of digestion or to a gangrenous section of bowel. A life-threatening intestinal obstruction is possible.
If the hernia can be easily pushed back in and there is little or no pain, a patient may wear a special supportive garment called a truss. This is usually a temporary measure until surgery can be performed.

Factors that increase your risk of complications:
Heart disease.
Obesity.
Prior unsuccessful hernia surgery.

Possible complications during and after surgery:
Bleeding.
Infection.
Recurrent hernia.
Sensory nerve injury.

Tests you may have to undergo:
Blood tests.
Chest X ray.

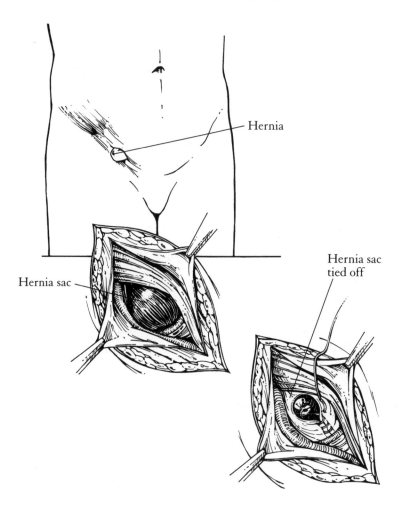

Hernia

Hernia sac

Hernia sac
tied off

EKG, if over sixty.
Physical examination.
Urinalysis.

Basic steps of the operation:
1. The surgery is usually done on an outpatient basis; anesthesia may be general or local.
2. An incision is made in the abdomen, usually in the groin area, at the site of the hernia.
3. The contents of the bulge are pushed back into place. The sac of abdominal lining itself is tied off and often removed.

4. The weakened area of tissue and muscle where the bulge oc-curred is strengthened by suturing or by a prosthetic fabric mesh that is sewn into the abdomen.
5. The incision is closed by sutures.
Duration: 45 to 90 minutes.

What to expect when it's over:
Patients usually leave the hospital the same day; pain in the area of the incision is treated by oral medication.
Return to work takes about 3 to 5 days.
Recovery takes about 2 to 3 weeks; heavy lifting should be avoided for a few months.
There is a small chance the hernia will recur.

OPEN PROSTATECTOMY/ TRANSURETHRAL RESECTION OF THE PROSTATE (TURP)/ PROSTATE GLAND PARTIAL REMOVAL

These related operations remove a portion of the prostate to relieve obstruction to the flow of urine. If the prostate has become enlarged, it can compress the urethra (urine channel) and change the shape of the bladder. The prostate gland produces the majority of the fluid that constitutes a man's ejaculate and that nourishes the sperm. After partial removal of the prostate, the volume of fluid may be normal, somewhat reduced, or almost nonexistent.

Part of the body operated on:
The prostate gland, through the abdomen or the penis.

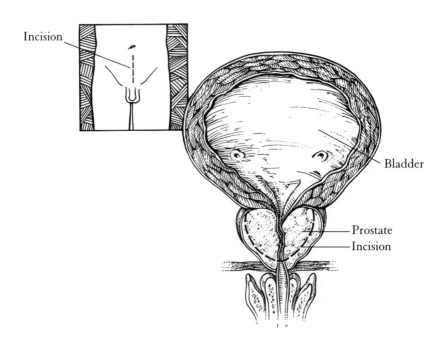

248

Reasons for having the operation:
Obstruction in the outflow of urine that cannot be controlled by medication.
Symptoms that become so severe that quality of life is affected.
Obstruction to the bladder is severe enough to jeopardize kidney function.
Symptoms include: weak urinary stream; hesitancy before urination starts; intermittent stream of urine that stops and starts; waking up at night to urinate; frequent urination during the day; feeling of urgency to urinate; incontinence (urination starts on its own); sensation that the bladder is not fully emptied.

What could happen if you don't have the operation:
Medications may diminish the intensity of the symptoms by shrinking or relaxing the tension of the prostate. These medications work on the muscle capsule of the prostate; once the muscle is relaxed, urine flows more easily through the prostate.

The condition may become so severe that any one of the following may occur:
Recurrent urinary-tract infections.
Recurrent and uncontrollable bleeding in the urine.
Impaired kidney function leading to a need for dialysis.
Inability to urinate.
Need for a permanent urinary catheter.
Permanent incontinence.
Death from complications of severe infection or renal failure.

Factors that increase your risk of complications:
Blood-clotting disorder.
Cardiovascular disease.
Kidney disease.
Untreated urinary-tract infection resulting in serious infection in the bloodstream.

Possible complications during and after surgery:
Bleeding.
Blood clots in the legs.

Damage to the nerves and blood vessels responsible for erection and causing loss of ability to have an erection.
Damage to the urinary sphincter resulting in urinary incontinence.
Dilution of blood from absorption of irrigation fluid during the operation.
Perforation of the bladder.

Tests you may have to undergo:
Blood tests.
Chest X ray.
Cystoscopy (inspection of the interior of the bladder).
EKG.
Urine culture.
Urodynamic study (similar to a stress test, but of the bladder).

Basic steps of the operation:
The operation is performed either through the penis or through the abdominal wall. The choice of approach depends on the size of the prostate. Very large prostates cannot be removed through the penis using the transurethral (TURP) procedure; these procedures must be performed by open prostatectomy.

Open Prostatectomy
1. The patient is anesthetized and the abdomen is opened by an incision above the pubic bone.
2. The bladder is exposed and opened.
3. The central portion of the prostate is scooped out to enlarge the urinary channel. There is no need to remove the entire gland because it would be very unusual for an obstruction to recur.
4. Bleeding is controlled with sutures and a catheter is placed in the bladder.
5. The bladder and incision are closed.
Duration: 2 to 3 hours.

Transurethral Resection of the Prostate (TURP)
1. The patient is anesthetized and a cystoscope (tube that provides a view of the bladder) is inserted through the urethra in the penis.

2. An instrument is passed through the tube to the prostate. Either by laser or electrocautery, the obstructing central prostate is scooped out in small sections.
3. The area is irrigated to wash away pieces of tissue; bleeding is stopped in surrounding blood vessels.
4. The scope is withdrawn and a catheter is inserted to drain urine.

Duration: 1 to 2 hours.

What to expect when it's over:

The catheter is removed 1 to 2 days after a TURP and in about 7 days following open surgery.

Once the catheter is removed, a patient may experience frequent urination, burning during urination, and some blood in the urine, especially at the beginning of urination. The symptoms gradually stop over a period of 1 to 12 weeks. The healthier the bladder was prior to surgery, the more quickly the bladder recovers. If surgery was delayed until symptoms were very severe, there can be a period of urinary incontinence.

In some instances, bladder relaxation medications may be necessary to aid in recovery.

If post-operative scarring were to occur and cause recurrent symptoms, it would do so within 6 months. It is very unusual for obstruction due to prostatic regrowth to recur.

RADICAL PROSTATECTOMY/ PROSTATE GLAND REMOVAL

This operation removes a cancerous prostate gland, an organ located beneath the bladder in men. The gland produces the majority of the fluid that constitutes a man's ejaculate and that nourishes the sperm. Following radical removal, there is no longer any ejaculate fluid.

Typically, the gland is the size of a lime or a lemon, though sometimes even normal glands can get as large as an orange or a grapefruit. (This may be due to cancer or a condition called BPH, benign prostatic hypertrophy.) It surrounds the urethra (the urine channel) like a doughnut with the urine channel running through the hole in the middle. The gland is very susceptible to the development of malignancy, and cancer of the prostate is the second most common form of cancer in men.

Part of the body operated on:
The prostate gland, through the lower abdomen, usually from the belly button to the pubic bone.

Reasons for having the operation:
To treat prostate cancer, if it has not spread beyond the prostate or metastasized to the lymph nodes or bone, by removing the entire gland. Cancer that has spread is not treated with surgery.

What could happen if you don't have the operation:
A patient could have another form of treatment such as radiation therapy.

If a patient chooses not to be treated, the cancer could spread and become incurable.

In some cases, the tumor is so small that it is not likely to spread during an elderly person's lifetime and that patient may choose not to have immediate therapy.

Factors that increase your risk of complications:
Other serious medical problems such as heart disease.

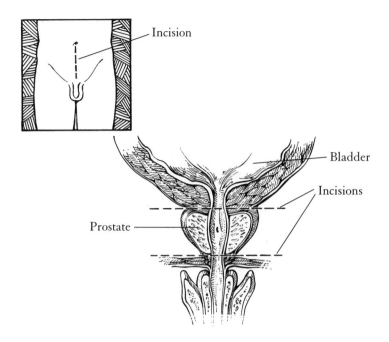

Possible complications during and after surgery:

Bleeding: The prostate gland sits in the pelvis beneath the bladder where it is surrounded by numerous large veins, which can sometimes bleed heavily. (Patients undergoing this operation are often asked to donate blood in advance to allow for transfusion of their own blood during the surgery.)

Impotence if nerves are cut.

Infection.

Leg and pelvic vein blood clots.

Tests you may have to undergo:

Blood tests.

Chest X ray.

Cystoscopy (inspection of the inside of the bladder and urethra by insertion of a scope).

EKG.

Prostate biopsy.

Rectal examination of the prostate.

Tests to assess whether cancer has spread include a CT scan, an MRI, and/or a bone scan.

Basic steps of the operation:
1. The patient is anesthetized and an incision is made in the lower abdomen, usually going from the belly button to the pubic bone.
2. The lymph nodes in the pelvis are removed and examined in the operating room by a pathologist using a process known as a frozen section.
3. The prostate gland is separated first from the muscles in the pelvis, then from the veins that drain the penis. Because these veins are so numerous and large, bleeding can result and must be controlled.
4. The urethral tube is separated from the prostate and cut above the urinary sphincter (valve that controls urine).
5. The prostate is then separated from the nerves and arteries that cause the penis to have an erection. The close proximity of these nerves and arteries to the penis means that a man's ability to get an erection following surgery can be affected.
6. The prostate is separated from the bladder. Once the prostate has been removed, the opening in the bladder must be closed and the bladder reattached to the urethral tube over a catheter that remains in the bladder for approximately 2 weeks.
7. A drain is placed in the wound to collect any leakage of urine or blood.
8. The incision is closed.

Duration: 4 to 5 hours.

What to expect when it's over:
In many cases, pain is minimal. Usually, a diet of clear liquids is started on the day of surgery or the next morning. A regular diet resumes as soon as a patient's body is ready to accept it.

The drain in the wound is usually removed in 2 to 3 days. The catheter in the bladder stays in for about 2 weeks.

Most patients are discharged from the hospital 2 to 3 days following the operation. They return in 2 weeks to the doctor's office to have the catheter removed and to discuss the pathology report. (The pathology report is usually available after one week.)

The risk of a serious incontinence problem (the daily need to wear a diaper or a pad) is related to the age of a patient and the health of the man's bladder. For men less than sixty years old with healthy bladders (no urgency to urinate and a forceful urinary stream), the risk is 1 percent. However, if a serious control problem results, there are steps that can be taken to restore urinary continence. Lesser incontinence (mild squirts) occur in 3 to 5 percent of men.

When the catheter is removed, a period of urinary incontinence (leakage) is expected. The degree of leakage decreases with time. Most patients regain control by about 3 months but in some instances, it may take as long as a year before full control returns. In the beginning, it may be necessary to wear an adult-sized diaper. As partial control returns, a pad can be worn inside underwear. Eventually, a patient wears only a light pad as a form of security to prevent leakage in a social setting. Once there is no further leakage, all types of pads become unnecessary.

Loss of some degree of erection ability is a very common problem, but the operation can be performed so that many men can regain their erectile ability. Greater than 95 percent of men less than sixty years old may regain their erection without the use of drugs such as Viagra. For older men or if erections have already weakened, the chance of recovery without medications is lessened.

Most patients can return to an active social life and nonphysical labor within 2 to 4 weeks. Exercise and physical exertion must be limited until full healing has taken place. This takes about 6 to 8 weeks. Attempts at sexual activity are usually resumed after 8 to 12 weeks.

If the pathology report indicates that cancer was confined to the prostate and that all of the surgical margins (edges of what was removed) are free of cancer, no further treatment is necessary. Because of microscopic spread beyond the prostate, some patients require post-operative radiation treatments. If this is required, it usually begins about 3 months after the operation.

17

Orthopedic Surgery

ARTHROPLASTY/
KNEE REPLACEMENT SURGERY

This operation replaces the knee joint with metal and plastic parts when bone and cartilage become severely worn.

Part of the body operated on:
The knee.

Reasons for having the operation:
Arthritis.
Pain in the knee that significantly affects movement.

What could happen if you don't have the operation:
The pain could increase.
Movement may become so impaired that a person may need a wheelchair.

Factors that increase your risk of complications:
Diabetes.
Emphysema.
History of blood clots.
Vascular disease.

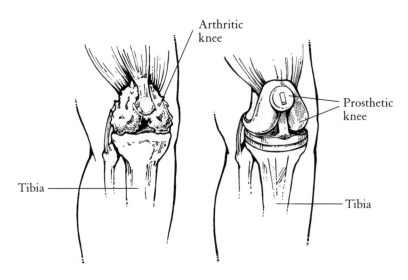

Arthritic
knee

Prosthetic
knee

Tibia

Tibia

Possible complications during and after surgery:
Blood clots.
Infection.
Knee stiffness.
Prosthetic failure over time.

Tests you may have to undergo:
Blood tests.
EKG.
X rays.

Basic steps of the operation:
1. Anesthesia is either regional (spinal or epidural) or general.
2. A long incision is made in the front of the knee. The surgeon moves aside the patella and reaches the joint.
3. The lower end of the thigh bone (femur) is shaped and holes are drilled into it to receive the metal replacement.
4. The upper end of the shin bone (tibia) is shaped and holes are cut into it to receive a plastic plate.
5. The back part of the knee cap (patella) is cut away to leave a flat surface. Small holes are drilled into it to receive a plastic button.

6. The prosthesis is cemented in place.
7. The incision is closed.
Duration: 4 hours.

What to expect when it's over:
A knee immobilizer (brace) for sleeping.
CPM (continuous passive motion) machine designed to bend the knee slowly and safely.
Intensive physical therapy.
A decrease in pain and increase in function.

Note: Long-term durability of parts is uncertain.

ARTHROSCOPY

In this type of surgery, a joint is inspected and may be repaired. The surgeon makes a very small incision and inserts an instrument called an arthroscope or endoscope. This illuminated tube's telescope-like features and a tiny camera allow the surgeon to see the affected area. It also projects the image of the inside of the joint onto a television monitor. The surgeon can pass instruments through the scope's channels to inflate, irrigate, and repair an area.

Part of the body operated on:
Most commonly the knee, but may also be done on the joints of the shoulder, elbow, wrist, hip, or ankle.

Reasons for having the operation:
Locking and catching in the joint.
Pain.
Swelling.

What could happen if you don't have the operation:
In most instances, persistence of these symptoms.

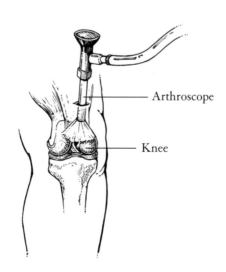

Arthroscope

Knee

Factors that increase your risk of complications:
Obesity.
Smoking.

Possible complications during and after surgery:
Bleeding.
Infection.
Phlebitis (swelling of a vein often accompanied by a blood clot).
Swelling.

Tests you may have to undergo:
Blood tests.
Chest X ray.
EKG (for people over forty years of age).

Basic steps of the operation:
1. Anesthesia may be general or local.
2. A very small incision is made in the skin.
3. An arthroscope is inserted. Air or a saline solution is injected to make the interior larger and easier to see.
4. The surgeon examines the bones, ligaments, cartilage, and membranes of the joint.
5. Through one or more additional small incisions, other instruments may be inserted to remove damaged tissue, repair small tears, or shave off areas of bone.

Duration: 45 minutes.

What to expect when it's over:
Hospital and recovery time is usually much less than in open (large incision, full view) surgery. With arthroscopy, patients are generally in the hospital no longer than 1 to 2 days; recovery is usually about 6 weeks. Exercise can be resumed immediately.

CARPAL TUNNEL SYNDROME REPAIR

A ligament (the transverse carpal ligament) covers the tunnel-like passage from the wrist to the hand, which contains tendons and a major nerve, called the median nerve. Lying like a band across the wrist, this ligament does not stretch. For a variety of reasons, including repetitive use of the wrist, the ligament can constrict the tendons and nerve underneath it. This surgery cuts through the ligament to open it up and release the pressure. A cut ligament does not impair movement since the ligament does not have any important functional purpose when using the wrist and hand.

Part of the body operated on:
The midsection of the palm, just beyond the wrist.

Reasons for having the operation:
Numbness in the fingers.
Pain in the wrist area.
Weakness or abnormal sensation in the hand.

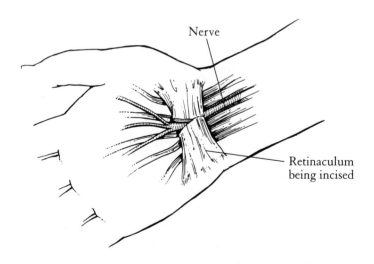

Nerve

Retinaculum
being incised

What could happen if you don't have the operation:
A splint may give temporary relief by preventing the movements
that aggravate the condition.
The symptoms would probably slowly worsen.
Permanent nerve damage may occur.

Factors that increase your risk of complications:
There are no real risk factors for this surgery.

Possible complications during and after surgery:
Failure to relieve the symptoms.
Nerve damage causing permanent numbness or loss of thumb
movement.

Tests you may have to undergo:
Possibly nerve-conduction studies (measurement of the speed of
electricity along the nerve).

Basic steps of the operation:
Surgery may be open or endoscopic. In endoscopic surgery, one or
two small incisions are made and visibility is provided into the interior by means of a viewing tube. In open surgery, the incision is
larger and there is direct vision of the operative area.

1. This surgery is done under local anesthesia. An incision is
   made in the skin of the palm.
2. The tight band over the carpal tunnel is cut to release it. Special
   care is taken not to cut any of the nearby nerves.
3. The ligament is left open; the skin of the palm is sewn closed.
Duration: ½ hour.

What to expect when it's over:
Normally, the wrist is immobilized with a bulky dressing (about an
inch thick going around the wrist) to allow the incision to heal for
a period of time that ranges from a few days to about 2 weeks.
During the time the wrist is immobilized, the patient should still be
using the fingers so that the hand does not become stiff.
There is an almost immediate and dramatic relief from pain caused
by the tight ligament. Some patients experience pillar pain, which

is a swelling in the base of the palm that can take 3 to 4 months to go away.

Return of strength in the wrist is slow and may not return to its preoperative levels. For example, patients may find it more difficult to grip and open the top of a jar. Some estimates show that by 6 weeks, about 50 percent of strength has returned.

DISCECTOMY/LUMBAR DISC SURGERY/ DISCECTOMY WITH FUSION

Discs are soft but tough tissues located in between each of the bones of the spine (vertebrae). The discs help link the vertebrae together allowing limited movement, so the spine is flexible but strong and stable. Discs also help keep vertebrae properly spaced apart so that the nerves coming from the inside of the spine have room to go out to other parts of the body. Since these nerves pass very close to the discs, they can be irritated if the disc is injured, worn out (degenerated), or torn (herniated). Extensive disc damage may weaken spinal linkage, allowing the spine to become painful and unstable.
Discectomy: *This operation removes disc material that is pressing on (compressing) nerves in the spine.*
Discectomy with fusion: *This operation not only removes disc material but also strengthens the spine by uniting (fusing) the bones together on either side of the damaged disc. Spinal fusion is done by bridging the vertebrae with bone; metal implants are often added to improve healing and speed recovery. (If you have a herniated disc in the upper spine/neck, you would have* cervical disc surgery, *which differs in several ways from lumbar surgery.)*

Part of the body operated on:
Lower back (lumbar spine).
Upper back (cervical spine).

Reasons for having the operation:
To relieve leg and back pain.
To prevent nerve damage.
To limit nerve damage that has already occurred.
To take pressure off spinal nerves and/or stabilize the spine if there is abnormal or painful movement.

What could happen if you don't have the operation:
If there is pain in the leg and/or back that is due to a herniated disc, but there is no nerve damage, the pain may be alleviated with physical therapy, exercise, and medication.

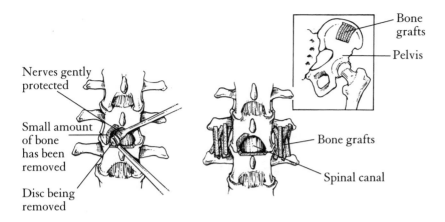

Nerves gently protected

Small amount of bone has been removed

Disc being removed

Bone grafts

Pelvis

Bone grafts

Spinal canal

If there is nerve damage, it may become permanent.

Immediate surgery may be needed, if there is any loss of bowel or bladder function.

Factors that increase your risk of complications:

Instability and weakness in the spine from pre-existing conditions such as arthritis, old injuries, or abnormal curvatures.

More than one disc is herniated or other spinal problems exist, like arthritis in the vertebrae.

Scarring from previous back surgery.

Smoking.

Possible complications during and after surgery:

Failure of bones to fuse.

Infection.

Nerve damage (very rare).

Scarring.

Tests you may have to undergo:

CT/myelogram: CT scan used with a dye to highlight nerves and where they go.

CT scan.

Discogram: X ray or CT scan with dye injected into the discs to determine which are damaged.

Donation of blood for lumbar decompression and fusion.

MRI.

Nerve tests: EMG (electromyogram) and SSEP (somatosensory evoked potential).

X rays.

Basic steps of the operation:

Discectomy:
1. General anesthesia is administered and a small incision is made in the lower back.
2. The soft tissues are gently pulled to the side (retracted) so that the vertebrae can be seen.
3. Small portions of bone and surrounding tissue are carefully removed so that the nerve and the disc can be safely seen.
4. The damaged portion of the disc is carefully removed.
5. The wound is closed.

Duration: 2 hours.

Lumbar Decompression and Fusion:

This operation is more extensive than discectomy alone.

Posterior Fusion (from the back of the body):
1. The patient is administered general anesthesia and an incision is made over the lower back.
2. Soft tissues are retracted to expose the vertebrae.
3. Bone, disc, and/or soft tissues, which are compressing nerves, are removed. A substantial amount of material can be removed since the spine will be stabilized (fused).
4. The vertebrae are prepared for fusion by scraping them to create a bleeding surface.
5. Bone graft (often taken from the pelvis) is placed along the prepared vertebrae.
6. Metal implants may be placed in the area as well.
7. The wound is closed.

Duration: 4 hours.

Anterior Fusion (from the front side):
1. The patient is administered general anesthesia and an incision is made over the lower abdomen or flank.
2. The abdominal contents are gently retracted so the front of the spine can be seen.

3. The injured disc is removed.
4. Bone graft and/or metal implants are placed.
5. The wound is closed.

Duration: 3½ to 4 hours.

What to expect when it's over:

Numbness and weakness is present, the severity of which depends on many factors, and may be difficult to predict.

After discectomy: Patients can get up soon after surgery (same day or next day). Pain often is better sooner and they can resume most activities after a few weeks.

After discectomy with fusion: It may take a few days until the patient can get up to walk. There may be discomfort in areas where bone graft was taken. Although back and leg pains are relieved within several weeks, 4 to 6 months are required to allow the fusion to start healing before full activity is allowed.

GANGLION CYST REMOVAL

This operation is done to remove a ganglion cyst, an abnormal growth of tissue, usually around a joint, but in some cases around a tendon. The cyst is filled with a clear fluid and most commonly appears on the back of the wrist (dorsal wrist, opposite the palm side). Less frequently, the cyst appears in other locations, like the palmar side of the wrist (this is more common in children).

Part of the body operated on:
The hand, on the back of the wrist; possibly other parts of the hand.

Reasons for having the operation:
The cyst continues to grow.
The cyst gets in the way or prevents the hand from moving properly.
Pain.

What could happen if you don't have the operation:
The cyst may go away on its own.
Symptoms could stay the same and if they're not bothersome, the cyst could be left alone.
Symptoms may get worse; a later operation could be more difficult because the cyst is larger.

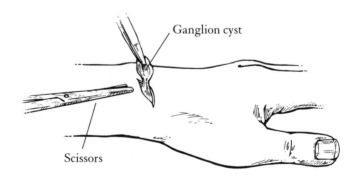

Ganglion cyst

Scissors

Factors that increase your risk of complications:
If the cyst has come back after a previous operation to remove it, scar tissues could make the surgery more difficult.

Possible complications during and after surgery:
Damage to major artery in the hand if the ganglion is near the palm.
Nerve injury and numbness.
Recurrence of cyst.
Unstable joint.

Tests you may have to undergo:
Possibly X rays.
Shining a light through the ganglion, since it is filled with clear fluid, to verify the nature of the mass.

Basic steps of the operation:
1. The surgery is usually done under regional anesthesia with sedation.
2. A tourniquet (a tight band inflated around the arm) temporarily cuts off the blood supply to the hand so there is no bleeding. Numbness of the area and sedation relieve any pressure or pain from the tourniquet.
3. The surgeon makes an incision directly over the ganglion.
4. The tissues between the skin and the ganglion are carefully spread apart to avoid cutting a nerve or artery.
5. The ganglion cyst is freed from surrounding tissues down to its base.
6. The ganglion is cut off at the base.
7. The skin of the hand is sewn closed.
Duration: 1 hour.

What to expect when it's over:
The area of the incision is covered with a bulky dressing (bandage wrapped around the wrist to the depth of about an inch) for 5 to 10 days.
During recovery, immediate movement of the wrist should be minimal, but the rest of the hand should be moved to prevent stiffness.

HIP REPLACEMENT SURGERY

The hip is a ball-and-socket joint. The ball-shaped top of the thigh bone (femur) glides inside the cup of the pelvic bone (acetabulum) when a person moves (as in walking). The cartilage that covers the ends of both of these bones makes the contact between them smooth. If this cartilage wears away, the ends of the bones rub against each other. The operation replaces the natural parts of the joint with artificial ones made of metal.

Part of the body operated on:
The hip.

Reasons for having the operation:
Relief from pain and stiffness that impair movement (may be caused by osteoarthritis or rheumatoid arthritis).
Fracture of the hip (femur) common in elderly females.

What could happen if you don't have the operation:
Anti-inflammatory medication can be tried to reduce arthritic symptoms.

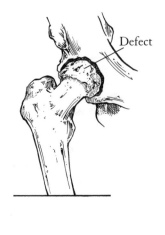
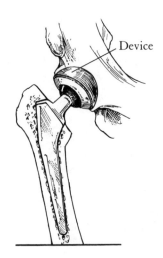

Some fractures may be able to heal with the help of metal screws and plates. Others require hip replacement surgery.

In the case of arthritis, if the condition does not improve, there will be continued pain and stiffness and reduced movement.

Factors that increase your risk of complications:
Other serious medical problems, including heart or lung disease.
Open sores or lesions that increase the risk of infection.

Possible complications during and after surgery:
Blood clot in the lungs or legs.
Hip dislocation.
Infection.
Nerve injury.

Tests you may have to undergo:
CT scan.
Donation of blood for hip replacements.
General medical clearance (blood tests, chest X ray, EKG).
MRI.
X rays of the hip.

Basic steps of the operation:
1. General or spinal anesthesia is administered.
2. An incision is made over the back of the hip. Muscles and tissues are cut or moved aside to expose the hip joint.
3. The thigh bone and the pelvic bone are separated. The socket in the pelvic bone is hollowed out further to provide space for the replacement cup. A metal shell with a plastic liner is inserted into the space.
4. The ball on the top of the thigh bone is removed and replaced with a metal ball that is attached to a metal stem. This stem is inserted into a canal in the thigh bone.
5. The replacement parts are locked in place, usually with a special cement that makes them adhere to the bone.
6. Any muscles or tendons that have been cut are repaired.
7. The incision is closed with staples or sutures.

Duration: 3 to 4 hours.

What to expect when it's over:

Physical therapy begins the first day after surgery. Two to 3 days later, patients are walking with the help of a walker. The usual length of hospitalization is 4 to 6 days. Some pain in the hip is usual in the first weeks and will ease as the area heals. Patients receive a blood thinner such as aspirin or coumadin to decrease the risk of blood clots.

In the first 6 weeks after surgery, patients are given the following instructions to prevent dislocation of the hip (the ball coming out of the socket):

Do not flex the hip higher than 90 degrees.
Do not cross the legs.
Sit on a high chair and high toilet seat.
Have someone put on your shoes and socks.
Sleep with a pillow between your legs.
Wear elastic stockings during the day to prevent swelling.
Continue exercises prescribed by a physical therapist.

Most of these changes can be modified substantially after 6 weeks when a person is fully ambulatory; however, precautions still need to be taken, including while sitting and bending.

ROTATOR CUFF REPAIR

This operation repairs torn or fraying muscles and tendons that allow the arm to rotate externally, raise up from the side (abduct), and be raised overhead. The tearing and fraying of these muscles may occur over time or be caused by accident or injury.

Part of the body operated on:
The four muscles that surround the shoulder and form the rotator cuff—the supraspinatus, infraspinatus, teres minor, and the subscapularis.

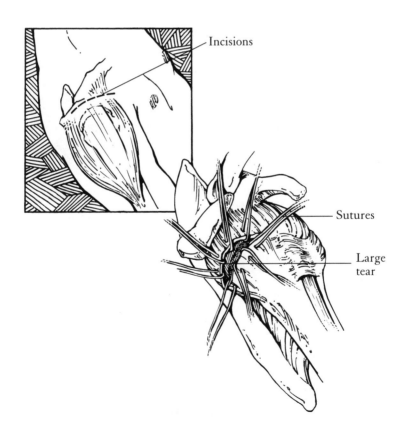

Incisions

Sutures

Large tear

Reasons for having the operation:
To keep the shoulder mobile.
To reduce pain.
To improve strength and function.

In some cases, symptoms can be managed through medication, re-
habilitative exercises, and rest. Surgery is often recommended if
the tear is severe enough to impair activities of daily living and
conservative treatment has failed.

What could happen if you don't have the operation:
Symptoms may worsen over time.
The tear could get bigger.
Possibility of subsequent muscle atrophy.
Range of motion and strength may decrease.
Early arthritis may develop.

Factors that increase your risk of complications:
Degree of trauma to the area.
Other chronic diseases or poor state of general health.
Poor rotator cuff tissue quality.

Possible complications during and after surgery:
Failure to improve function of the shoulder.
Infection.
Nerve injury.
Pain.

Tests you may have to undergo:
Blood tests.
MRI.
Physical exam that includes testing strength and range of motion.
X rays.

Basic steps of the operation:
The surgery may be either arthroscopic, arthroscopically assisted
(mini-open), or open. The type of surgery is based on length, width,
and depth of the tear and the number of muscles involved. If the

tear is small or incomplete, arthroscopic surgery may be done. Anesthesia is administered with a regional block unless medically contraindicated.

Arthroscopic:
1. After the patient has been anesthetized, 2 to 4 incisions of less than an inch are made in the shoulder. An arthroscope, or illuminated viewing instrument, is inserted and the area is examined. A saline solution is injected into the area to distend it for better viewing.
2. The surgeon debrides (repairs) fraying areas of the tendon and surrounding structures with a motorized shaver.
3. The incisions are closed.
Duration: 2 hours.

Mini-open:
This surgery combines the techniques of arthroscopy with a small open incision for the repair of the rotator cuff. It is usually done with partial-thickness and small full-thickness tears that need suturing.

Open:
1. This surgery is used with large full-thickness tears. The patient is anesthetized and an incision of about 3 to 4 inches is made in the deltoid muscle to expose the rotator cuff.
2. A small amount of acromion (bone) is often removed in both this and the other types of surgery to relieve impingement (muscle wears up against the bone when lifting the arm overhead, for example).
3. Tears are then repaired by suturing.
4. The incision is closed.
Duration 2 to 3 hours.

What to expect when it's over:
Immediately after surgery, pain is controlled by the regional nerve block, which lasts for several hours. Pain may vary according to which technique was used. Open procedures are often associated with more pain and narcotic medication is used during the hospital stay. Following arthroscopic surgery, the patient goes home the same day and is given oral pain medication.

The arm is in a sling for about 2 days after arthroscopic surgery; about 10 days after mini-open surgery; and about 4 to 6 weeks after open surgery.

Physical therapy is started immediately to regain range of motion and strength. It lasts for several months and the patient is able to do much of it independently.

Eighty-five to 95 percent of patients have significant improvement in function; more than 90 percent have pain relief.

SCOLIOSIS SURGERY

Scoliosis means abnormal lateral (sideways) curvature of the spine. Most people with scoliosis never need surgery. When necessary, scoliosis surgery prevents the condition from becoming worse by fusing (joining) two or more separate vertebrae together into a single, longer bone in the curved part of the spine.

Special metal rods are placed along the spine to hold it in place while the bones heal and become fused. In some cases two operations are needed, one from the front of the spine and the other from the back.

Part of the body operated on:
The thoracic (upper) and/or the lumbar (lower) spine.

Reasons for having the operation:
To treat pain, severe deformity, or imbalance.
To prevent curvature from getting worse.
To prevent onset or worsening of nerve damage.

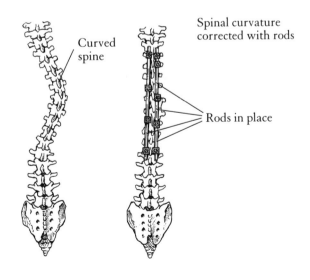

Curved spine

Spinal curvature corrected with rods

Rods in place

What could happen if you don't have the operation:
In children:
If the curvature is small, less than 20 degrees, it may not progress and no treatment is necessary. Careful follow-up is recommended.

Growing children with larger curves (20 to 40 degrees) may need a brace to direct growth and prevent the curve from getting worse. The brace is custom-molded from firm plastic and covers much of the torso.

Large curves (greater than 40 to 50 degrees) cannot be controlled with a brace, are likely to get worse, and generally require surgery.

Adults:
Slight scoliosis does not require treatment.

Larger curves, with symptoms of back and leg pain, numbness, or weakness, can be treated with physical therapy, medication, and a brace before surgery is considered.

Factors that increase your risk of complications:
Prior surgery.
Severe deformity.
Smoking.

Possible complications during and after surgery:
Failure of spine to fuse (adults).
Infections.
Nerve damage.

Tests you may have to undergo:
Blood tests.
CT scan.
MRI.
Myelogram.
X rays.

Basic steps of the operation:
Scoliosis surgery usually requires a blood transfusion. When possible, patients should donate their own blood. In addition, a "cell-saver" machine is frequently used to recycle blood during surgery.

1. The patient is administered general anesthesia.
2. Patient is positioned face down (prone) if the approach is from the back (posterior surgery); on the side (anterior) for approach from the front (anterior surgery).
3. When indicated, monitoring of the nerves is done by means of electrical signals from leads attached to the patient; this continues throughout the operation to make sure the nerves are all right.
4. The spine is exposed. If the approach is posterior, the incision is made in the middle of the back. If it is anterior, the incision is made on the side of the body, over the chest, or the abdomen. A rib is often removed and can be used as a bone graft. Sometimes the anterior procedure can be done through a "scope."
5. The outer surface (cortex) of the vertebrae being treated is intentionally scratched or roughened so it bleeds (decorticated).
6. These decorticated surfaces are then bridged together by bone grafts, which are taken from the pelvis or rib. These bone grafts span from one vertebra to the next. They are not actually attached to the vertebrae, but are held in place by a tight envelope of connective tissue.
7. Special metal screws, hooks, and/or cables are attached to several different vertebrae. Together these devices serve as anchors, connected by metal rods. They help hold the vertebrae in the correct position so that the vertebrae can fuse together. The metal implants are usually left in place indefinitely.
8. In certain situations, corrections of the curvature can also be improved by removing discs (discectomy) and/or by cutting the spinal bone (osteotomy).
9. If nerve monitoring suggests there might be a question about nerve function, a "wake-up test" can be done. General anesthesia is reduced so that the patient can be asked to move feet and toes. Once this is done, the regular level of anesthesia is resumed.
10. A chest tube may be put in place if the anterior approach involved the chest.
11. The incision is closed.

Duration: 4 to 5 hours.

In some cases, both front and back surgery is needed. The second surgery may be done the same day, or a few days later.

What to expect when it's over:

Most patients can get out of bed within 2 or 3 days. Pain is controlled by narcotic medication. The hospital stay is 2 weeks.

Some patients may need to wear a brace for 3 to 4 months after surgery.

Most activities can be resumed once the fusion has healed. Contact sports should be avoided for the rest of the patient's life.

18

Reproductive Surgery

BILATERAL TUBAL LIGATION (BTL)/ STERILIZATION

This operation cuts or obstructs the fallopian tubes, the organs where the eggs are fertilized by sperm. After the operation sperm can no longer encounter an egg and pregnancy is not possible.

Part of the body operated on:
The fallopian tubes, through the abdomen.

Reasons for having the operation:
To prevent pregnancy permanently. It is usually done when a woman is sure she does not want children in the future and would prefer not to use other methods of contraception. In rare cases, a woman may have the surgery because she has an illness that would put her life in grave danger if she became pregnant.
It is very important to have presurgical counseling to review all other options for contraception before making a decision that renders a woman permanently sterile.

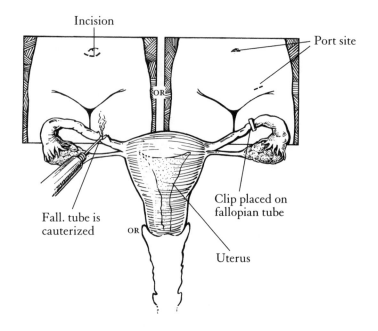

Incision
Port site
Fall. tube is cauterized
OR
Clip placed on fallopian tube
Uterus

What could happen if you don't have the operation:
You could use alternative forms of contraception: birth-control pills, IUD, diaphragm, or condoms.

Factors that increase your risk of complications:
Hernia that contains abdominal organs.
Infection in the abdomen.
Intestines that are distended due to bowel obstruction or malfunction.
Obesity.
Previous abdominal surgeries.
Problems with blood clotting.
Severe cardiac or respiratory disease.

Possible complications during and after surgery:
Bleeding or infection. The risk of such complications is very small, but slightly higher if the surgery is done in the postpartum period, since blood vessels are enlarged during pregnancy and the pelvic organs are being manipulated to a greater degree than if the sterilization is done well after delivery.
Sterilization failure: About 2 to 4 women out of 1,000 who undergo this procedure later become pregnant. Of the women who become

pregnant, there is the risk that the pregnancy is ectopic (in the tubes), which can lead to internal hemorrhaging and may become life-threatening if not detected early.

Tests you may have to undergo:
Blood tests.
Complete gynecological exam with a Pap smear.

Basic steps of the operation:
Postpartum open surgery (shortly after the vaginal delivery of a child): The uterus is still enlarged at this time and it is easier to access the fallopian tubes at the level of the umbiculus. If a woman is having a cesarean section, the tubal ligation can be performed during that operation.
1. A horizontal incision of about 1 to 2 inches is made just below the navel, after anesthesia has been administered.
2. The abdominal tissue is cut and separated until the uterus is reached.
3. The tubes are identified and pulled up and out through the incision.
4. Most commonly, a segment of tube is cut out. Other methods to block the tubes include: cautery (burning a section of the tube); constricting the tube with a tight band; placing a plastic or metal clip to obstruct the tube; removing both tubes completely.
5. The abdominal incision is closed.
Duration: 30 minutes.

Laparoscopic sterilization:
1. General anesthesia is administered and a very small incision is made in the navel and the laparoscope (viewing tube) is inserted.
2. The surgeon injects carbon dioxide gas to expand the area, making the organs visible through the viewing tube.
3. One or two additional instruments needed for the procedure are placed through small incisions in the lower abdomen.
4. The tubes are cut or obstructed by one of the methods described in step 4 of *postpartum open surgery.*
5. The instruments are removed, the gas is evacuated, and the incisions are closed.
Duration: 1 hour.

What to expect when it's over:
Pain or discomfort is typically alleviated with Tylenol or a similar product.

Most women are able to return to normal functioning within 24 to 36 hours.

Sexual activity can resume in about 1 week.

Reversal of sterilization is possible in some cases. If an adequate length of tube remains, pregnancy rates after a reversal can be up to 50 to 70 percent. If a pregnancy does occur, there is a 10 to 20 percent chance that it would be an ectopic or tubal pregnancy, which can be life-threatening. This is treated by surgically removing the tubal pregnancy and usually the entire fallopian tube. If both tubes are surgically removed, the only option for future child-bearing is through in vitro fertilization.

GYNECOLOGIC LAPAROSCOPY

Examination of the female pelvic area by means of a long, slender, telescope-like instrument inserted through a puncture-like incision. The surgeon is able to view the interior and the pelvis, investigate causes of problems, and, in many cases, treat them at the same time.

Part of the body operated on:
Abdomen and internal organs including: uterus, fallopian tubes, ovaries, appendix, and bladder supports.

Reasons for having the operation:
Ectopic pregnancy (fetus develops outside of the uterus).
Endometriosis (small pieces of the lining of the uterus adhere to organ walls and may grow into cysts).
Infertility.
Ovarian cysts or fibroids (benign tumors of the uterus).
Pelvic adhesions (abnormal scar tissue that adheres to the organs and causes distortion and pain).

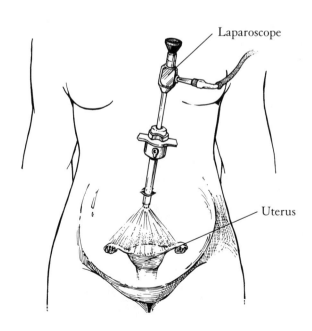

Laparoscope

Uterus

Sterilization (tubal ligation).
Unexplained pain or infection.

What could happen if you don't have the operation:
Conditions that cannot be diagnosed by other means may go untreated, such as cysts, fibroids, and other adhesions.
Alternative is more extensive and invasive surgery such as an open
laparotomy for diagnostic purposes.

Factors that increase your risk of complications:
Heart/lung disease.
Obesity.
Prior surgery of the abdomen.

Possible complications during and after surgery:
Hernia.
Infection.
Injury or perforation of the bowel, bladder, or ureter (tube that car-
ries urine from the kidney to the bladder) that might require ad-
ditional surgery to correct.
Laceration of blood vessels.

Tests you may have to undergo:
Blood tests.
Sonogram (ultrasound scanning in which sound waves are used to
create an image of the interior reproductive organs).
Urinalysis.

Basic steps of the operation:
1. The procedure is usually done on an outpatient basis with either general or local anesthesia.
2. Carbon dioxide gas is pumped into the abdomen from a hollow
   needle that is inserted through the navel. The resulting infla-
   tion of the abdomen enables the surgeon to get a better view of
   the internal organs.
3. An incision of about a half-inch is made in the abdomen at the
   navel. The laparoscope is inserted through it to view the reproductive area. If it is necessary to follow up with surgical proce-

dures, another very small incision is made at the pubic hairline for the insertion of instruments.

4. The surgeon can perform several different treatments including: removal of abnormal scar tissue; destruction of growths caused by endometriosis; injection of a dye to see if a fallopian tube is blocked; possible removal of an ectopic pregnancy; treatment of cysts and tumors; tubal sterilization by clip; suspension of bladder; cauterization of a ring (tissue obstructing a fallopian tube); removal of fibroids; removal of uterus.

5. The gas is released from the abdomen and the incisions are closed with sutures.

Duration: 2 hours.

What to expect when it's over:

Oral pain medication is prescribed for pain at the site of the incision; pressure or irritation from the gas could cause pain for 1 to 2 days. There may be a small amount of vaginal bleeding for a few days. Patients can usually resume normal activities within 1 to 2 days.

HYSTERECTOMY

Removal of the uterus and, usually, the cervix.

Part of the body operated on:
Abdomen or vagina; uterus and cervix.

Reasons for having the operation:
Fibroids (benign tumors).
Cancer of the uterus, cervix, or ovaries.
Endometriosis (pieces of tissue in the lining of the uterus become
  displaced, move to other parts of the abdomen, and cause pain) if
  it cannot be successfully treated by other means.
Precancerous conditions in the uterine area.
Severely prolapsed uterus (the uterus stretches and sags into the
  vagina).
Unusually heavy menstrual bleeding or pain.

What could happen if you don't have the operation:
If a patient has cancer, it could become life-threatening.
Symptoms of benign fibroids, including pelvic pain, bleeding, or
  pain during sexual intercourse, could become worse.

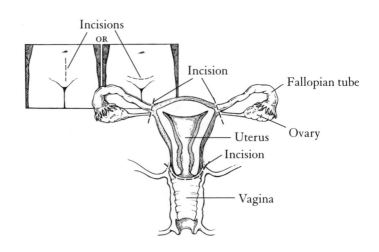

Factors that increase your risk of complications:
Chronic disease.
High blood pressure.
Obesity.
Poor nutrition.
Smoking.

Possible complications during and after surgery:
Bleeding.
Blood clots in the legs.
Infection.

Tests you may have to undergo:
Blood tests.
CT scan.
Diagnostic laparoscopy.
MRI.
X rays.

Basic steps of the operation:
1. The operation is done under general or regional anesthesia. Either an abdominal incision or a vaginal approach is used.
2. For the abdominal operation, an incision is made, usually about 5 inches long in a horizontal cut across the lower abdomen. An abdominal incision gives more visibility to the surgeon and is often used when there are large tumors. This procedure may cause more discomfort in recovery and a visible scar, although it is usually made as close to the top of the pubic hairline as possible.
3. For the vaginal operation, the incision is made from inside the vagina. There is no external scar, but the vagina is slightly shortened.
4. In both types of surgery, the uterus is separated from the fallopian tubes, which are tied off. (In some cases, the ovaries and fallopian tubes are also removed.) The uterus is separated from the vagina, which is stitched closed.
5. The abdominal incisions are sewn in a layered closure.
Duration: 2 hours.

What to expect when it's over:

A patient is usually hospitalized for 3 to 4 days; she can generally walk on the second day.

The first night, the patient has a urinary catheter; an IV may remain in place for 2 to 3 days.

Medication is prescribed for post-operative pain, which is usually greatest in the area of the incision.

Recovery takes about 4 weeks, during which time a patient can gradually resume activities. Lifting should be avoided during the first 2 weeks.

Sexual intercourse can be resumed in about 6 to 8 weeks.

The patient no longer has menstrual periods and cannot become pregnant.

If the surgery is done before menopause has begun, a patient may experience the symptoms of menopause and choose to consider hormone-replacement therapy.

Some patients may experience emotional and psychological difficulty in the aftermath of this surgery. Patients may find one-on-one counseling with a qualified therapist helpful.

19

Transplantation Surgery

HEART TRANSPLANTATION

Replacing a patient's own heart with a heart from another person.

Part of the body operated on:
The heart, through the chest.

Reasons for having the operation:
The patient's own heart is too diseased to keep him alive and its problems cannot be treated by other medical or surgical means. There are two main problems that result in the need for transplantation:

Irreversible damage to the heart from hardening of the arteries and multiple heart attacks.
Heart muscle disease in which the heart cannot contract normally because of damage to the muscle cells.

Other less common reasons for having a transplant include: abnormalities of the heart valves, congenital heart defects, or heart tumors.

What could happen if you don't have the operation:
The patient is at a high risk of dying.

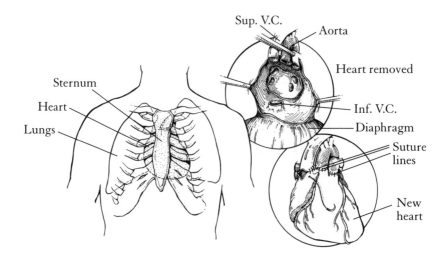

Factors that increase your risk of complications:
Active infections.
Age: transplants are generally done on patients under the age of
sixty-five.
Alcoholism or drug abuse.
High blood pressure in the lungs (pulmonary hypertension).
Obesity.
Recent cancer.
Smoking.

Possible complications during and after surgery:
Bleeding.
Death.
Failure of the heart to function properly.
Infection.
Problems in the organs to which the heart pumps blood, including
the lungs, liver, or kidneys.
Rejection of the heart by the body's immune system.
Stroke.

Tests you may have to undergo:
Extensive pre-operative evaluation to see if heart transplantation is

the best option and to uncover any other organ problems or disease. Tests include:

Complete physical exam, including EKG; blood, urine, and skin tests; X rays; possibly cardiac catheterization.
Full dental exam with X rays to rule out any mouth infection.
Neurological exam and brain tests if indicated by patient's condition.
Physical-therapy examination to assess joint motion, muscle strength, and ability to participate in routine exercises.
Psychiatric evaluation to review emotional function and ability to cope with stress.

Basic steps of the operation:
1. When a suitable donor becomes available: recipient match is identified based on blood type, weight, geographical location, and severity of illness. A medical team rushes to the location of the donor heart, examines the heart, places it in a special cold solution to keep it alive outside the body, and transports it to the medical center where the patient is ready to receive it. Time is of the essence: a heart can be disconnected from a person for only about 4 hours before it begins to lose its ability to work properly upon reconnection.
2. The recipient/patient is anesthetized. A Foley catheter is inserted to drain the bladder.
3. The chest is cleaned with an antiseptic. An incision is made over the sternum (breastbone) and the bone divided to allow access to all parts of the heart. The patient is connected to the heart-lung bypass machine, which circulates the blood and provides oxygen to it.
4. The surgeon opens the pericardium, the sac that contains the heart, and removes the diseased heart. Simultaneously, the donor heart is brought to the operating room.
5. The surgeon carefully fits the new heart into place and sews it to the major blood vessels.
6. The new heart begins to function and blood flow is reestablished. Once the heart is beating, the patient is taken off the heart-lung bypass machine.

7. Tubes are placed in the chest for drainage of fluids during recovery. Pacing wires are brought out of the chest cavity through the skin surface in case there's a need for electrical pacing. The sternum is closed with stainless-steel wires and the fatty tissues and skin are closed with absorbable sutures.
Duration: 5 hours.

What to expect when it's over:

The patient is taken to the intensive-care unit where he regains consciousness. He has a breathing tube in his mouth and throat and can't talk, eat, or drink. When the patient awakens, the tube is removed. Intravenous lines in the arms and neck provide fluids and medication. The catheter remains in the bladder. Wires on the chest monitor the new heart. These tubes and wires remain in place as long as they're necessary. Some will be removed as early as the first day after surgery.

Immunosuppressive medications are begun and adjusted. Patient remains on these medications permanently.

If there are no post-operative complications, the patient can leave the ICU as early as 1 to 2 days after the operation and go to a regular hospital room. There the patient is encouraged to do exercises in bed, perform breathing exercises, cough, and walk. These may cause pain at the site of the incision and the patient is instructed on how to reduce pain. Walking begins as soon as possible after surgery—if all goes well, in 7 to 10 days.

Time of discharge is based on the rate of healing, the result of cardiac biopsies to monitor rejection, and the ability to tolerate medicines.

It takes about 8 weeks for the bones and tissues of the chest to heal. Most patients resume driving about 3 months after the operation and return to work within 6 months. Patients should discuss with their physician the pace of their return to other lifestyle activities and their resumption of exercise and sexual activity.

Recipients need to take immunosuppressive medication to prevent rejection for the rest of their lives.

KIDNEY TRANSPLANTATION

The kidneys are two organs about 4 or 5 inches long behind the abdominal cavity, on either side of the spine. One of their main jobs is to filter out and secrete waste products from the blood. If a patient has kidney disease that prevents the kidneys from functioning normally (renal failure), that purification process can be done through a mechanical process called dialysis.

In one method, the patient is connected several times a week (for 3 to 4 hours each time) to a dialysis machine that removes waste products from the blood and returns the purified blood to the body. In the other technique, the patient puts specialized fluid into the abdominal cavity several times a day by means of a permanent catheter. The fluid mixes with waste products filtered from the blood into the abdominal cavity and is then drained out into a bag, which is emptied 4 times per day.

Even with dialysis, a person's general state of health and quality of life becomes increasingly impaired over time. A kidney transplant is considered to be the best and safest solution for long-term treatment of renal failure.

The function of the diseased kidneys, which are not removed unless they cause infection or high blood pressure, is supplemented by a single healthy kidney. The new kidney comes from a person who has just died (cadaver) or from a living person who is willing to donate a kidney. It is necessary to find a kidney that is compatible with the blood type of the patient. If the kidney is from a cadaver, the operation has to be performed on an emergency basis. If it is donated from a living person, the surgery can be planned and the donor and recipient operations are usually done at the same time in adjourning operating rooms.

Part of the body operated on:

Lower abdomen, on the right or left side, to place the kidney in the pelvis with blood vessels of the new kidney connected to the artery and vein that goes to the leg.

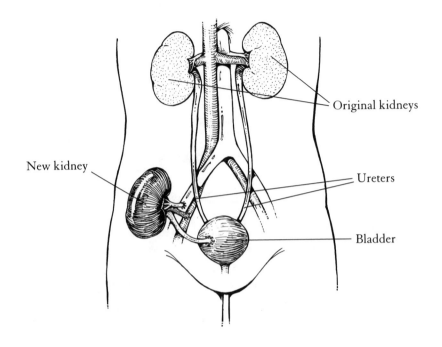

Reasons for having the operation:
The failure of a person's natural kidneys.

What could happen if you don't have the operation:
Patient would stay on dialysis as long as possible barring major complications.

Factors that increase your risk of complications:
Diabetes.
Heart problems.
Poor circulation in the legs.
Smoking.
Stroke.

Possible complications during and after surgery:
Abdominal pain.
Bleeding.
Constipation.
Infection.

Kidney rejection.
Problems with arteries and veins going to the leg.
Slow recovery of function of the transplanted kidney.

Tests you may have to undergo:
Bladder and blood vessel tests in older patients.
Blood tests to determine genetic makeup.
Cardiac stress test if older than forty years of age.
Chest X ray.
Upper and lower GI series.

Basic steps of the operation:
1. The operation is done under general anesthesia.
2. A skin incision of about 8 to 10 inches is made in the lower abdomen.
3. The new kidney is placed just outside the abdominal cavity, in a different location from the old kidneys, usually above the groin in the pelvis, near the bladder. The artery and vein of the new kidney is sewn to the patient's artery and vein that go to the legs.
4. The ureter (tube that carries urine) of the new kidney is attached to the patient's bladder.
5. The incision is sewn closed.
Duration: 2½ to 5 hours.

What to expect when it's over:
Abdominal discomfort or pain lasts about 1 week. The hospital stay is usually about 3 to 5 days.
The kidney may begin to produce urine either immediately or in several days or even weeks later. Once the kidney is functioning well, there is no further need for dialysis. If the kidney does not function promptly, dialysis may be briefly needed after the operation.
There is a rare chance that the kidney may never function, or be rejected during the operation or shortly thereafter. The patient would then need to return to dialysis and to have a second transplant operation when a kidney became available. The kidney may undergo a rejection episode at any time but especially in the first

three months. This can usually be reversed with medications, allowing the kidney to continue to work.

In the long run, the likelihood that a kidney taken from a cadaver will continue to work for 10 years is about 50 percent. If the kidney is from a living donor, it is about 80 to 85 percent.

Recipients need to take immunosuppressive medication to prevent rejection for the rest of their lives. In some cases, patients experience side effects from the drugs, including susceptibility to infections. Short-term effects may include weight gain, growth of body hair with some drugs, headaches, and high blood pressure. Rarely, transient diabetes may occur while some patients may develop abdominal cramps and diarrhea that disappear with the lowering of doses.

LUNG TRANSPLANTATION

Replacement of diseased lung (may be one or both lungs) with new lung(s).

Part of the body operated on:
The chest.

Reasons for having the operation:
Chronic obstructive pulmonary disease (COPD). Symptoms include shortness of breath, coughing, wheezing, and weakness. Air does not flow normally in the lungs. A patient may have damaged air sacs that exchange oxygen for carbon dioxide in the lungs (emphysema); narrow and inflamed airways characterized by attacks of breathlessness (chronic asthma); or inflamed, narrowed, and obstructed airways clogged by large amounts of mucus (chronic bronchitis). Some people have more than one of these conditions.
Pulmonary fibrosis (scarring and thickening of lung tissue).
Cystic fibrosis (chronic lung infections due to an inherited disease).

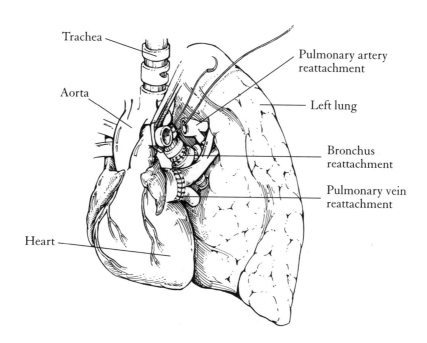

Pulmonary hypertension (resistance to blood flow through the lungs and increased pressure in the arteries supplying them).

What could happen if you don't have the operation:
Patients may have respiratory or heart failure leading to death. Only patients who are estimated to have no more than 2 years to live are considered as candidates for a transplant.

Factors that increase your risk of complications:
Active infection.
Advanced age.
Previous surgery of the lungs or heart.

Possible complications during and after surgery:
Failure of the transplanted lung to function.
Infection.
Pneumonia.

Tests you may have to undergo:
Chest X ray.
CT scan.
Evaluation of lifestyle and psychological status.
Extensive blood work.
Heart catheterization.
Lung scan.

Basic steps of the operation:
The lung from a donor is flushed with a cold solution and packed in an ice water bath. Its temperature is kept very low so that it does not require oxygen.

1. The patient is administered general anesthesia. If one lung is available for breathing, a breathing tube is used; otherwise, the patient is connected to a heart-lung machine, which does the work of breathing during the operation.
2. An incision is made on the side of the chest. If both lungs are being removed, one lung is done at a time.
3. The diseased lung is cut from the heart and the trachea.

4. The new lung is placed in the patient's chest and sewn to the heart and the trachea.
5. The incision is sewn closed.

Duration: 6 hours.

What to expect when it's over:
Hospital stay is about 2 to 3 weeks. The patient remains on a respirator for 1 to 2 days.

Pain is controlled for 5 to 7 days after surgery with narcotic medication that is either introduced by epidural catheter or intravenously.

Patients must remain on immunosuppressive drugs to prevent organ rejection.

It may be 3 to 6 months before patients make a full return to normal activities.

20

Vascular Surgery

ABDOMINAL AORTIC ANEURYSM REPAIR

The aorta—the long artery that goes from the heart to the groin—may have a weak segment in its wall that becomes distended from the pressure of blood flowing through it. In the surgery that repairs this condition, the site of the ballooning, called an aneurysm, is replaced by a synthetic tube.

Part of the body operated on:
The abdomen, extending down to the lower portion where the aorta divides to form the two iliac arteries.

Reasons for having the operation:
To prevent rupture of the artery wall.

What could happen if you don't have the operation:
If the aneurysm ruptured, it could cause death.

Factors that increase your risk of complications:
Heart or lung disease.

Possible complications during and after surgery:
Bleeding.
Death.

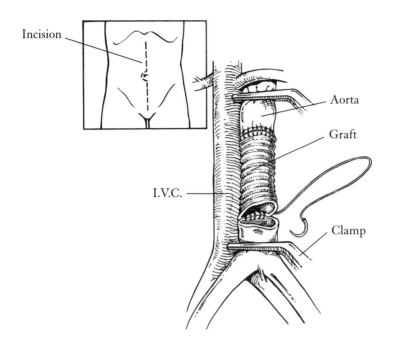

Heart attack.
Kidney failure.
Stroke.

Tests you may have to undergo:
Blood tests.
Chest X ray.
CT scan of abdomen.
EKG.
Ultrasound of aorta.

Basic steps of the operation:
1. The patient is administered general anesthesia.
2. The abdomen is opened, usually by an incision that extends from below the breastbone to the pubic area.
3. The aneurysm is removed and replaced with the artificial blood vessel, which is sewn to the aorta above and below the site of the aneurysm. This part of the surgery must be per-

formed quickly because the blood flow to the lower body is cut off while the graft is securely connected to the aorta.
4. Blood flow resumes through the artificial artery.
5. The abdomen is closed by sutures or staples.
Duration: 4 hours.

What to expect when it's over:

Recovery begins in the intensive-care unit; the hospital stay usually lasts about 7 days. Pain from the incision is controlled by medication.

Recovery may last several weeks at home; it is normal to feel tired and weak. Return to normal activities is slow. Lifting, or other moves that put stress on the abdomen, should be avoided for 6 weeks.

CAROTID ARTERY ENDARTERECTOMY

*This operation removes plaque (fatty tissue) that can build up
in the carotid arteries that lead from the heart to the brain.*

Part of the body operated on:
The neck.

Reasons for having the operation:
To enhance blood flow to the head.
To prevent a stroke.

What could happen if you don't have the operation:
The opening in the artery could become so narrow that the blood
supply to the brain would be seriously reduced.
A stroke could occur resulting in disability or death.

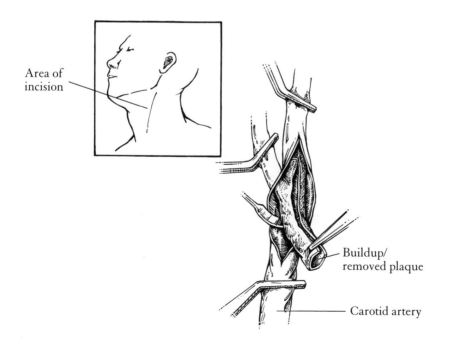

Area of
incision

Buildup/
removed plaque

Carotid artery

Factors that increase your risk of complications:
Other forms of heart or lung disease.

Possible complications during and after surgery:
Bleeding or infection (rarely).
Stroke.

Tests you may have to undergo:
Blood tests.
Chest X ray.
EKG.
Possibly an angiogram (an X ray that uses injected dye to show the interior of the arteries).
Ultrasound exam of the carotid artery.

Basic steps of the operation:
1. The surgery is done under general anesthesia.
2. A 3-inch incision is made on the side of the neck and the artery is exposed.
3. A small incision may also be made on the thigh to harvest a vein, which will be used to reconstruct the carotid artery.
4. The surgeon removes the plaque with a specialized instrument to clean out the artery.
5. The incisions in the arteries and the neck are closed with sutures.

Duration: 1½ to 2 hours.

What to expect when it's over:
Hospital stay is usually 1 to 2 days. Most patients can resume normal activities within 7 to 10 days.
Mild headache can occur due to the restoration of blood flow to the brain. It usually goes away in a few days.

PERIPHERAL VASCULAR DISEASE BYPASS

An operation to enable blood to flow around a blockage in the artery in the leg. A plastic tube or a vein from another part of the body is sewn onto the artery at points above and below the blockage; blood flow is redirected through the new passageway.

Part of the body operated on:
The leg.

Reasons for having the operation:
Atherosclerosis: hardening of the arteries due to a buildup of material called plaque on the inner wall of the artery.
Claudication: the narrowing of the artery due to plaque buildup; blood flow is reduced and after a short walk, the leg cramps or becomes tired.

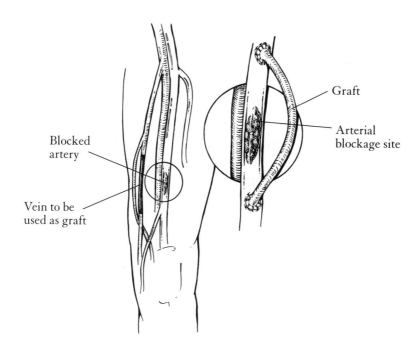

Graft

Arterial
blockage site

Blocked
artery

Vein to be
used as graft

What could happen if you don't have the operation:
Continuation of poor circulation and symptoms including pain in the affected limb, inability to walk far, and ulcers on the feet.
In severe cases, gangrene occurs in the feet or toes and a limb may be lost.

Factors that increase your risk of complications:
Diabetes.
Heart disease.
High blood pressure.
High cholesterol level.
Smoking.

Possible complications during and after surgery:
Bleeding or blood clots.
Heart attack.
Poor drainage of the wound and infection.

Tests you may have to undergo:
Blood tests.
Chest X ray.
ECG or a stress test.
EKG.
Tests to measure blood flow including blood pressure in the legs and imaging of the artery through sound waves.

Basic steps of the operation:
1. The patient is given general anesthesia or an epidural injection. Blood-thinning medication prevents clotting.
2. Incisions are made on the calf or thigh above and below the site of the blockage and the artery is examined.
3. Several small incisions are made to obtain veins to be used for the bypass; in other cases, plastic tubes manufactured to medical specifications are used.
4. The tube or vein is sewn to the section of artery with a good pulse and is passed under the skin to meet the artery where the pulse is poor. Blood then flows through this bypass.

5. The blocked section is usually left in the leg; in some cases, it may be cleaned out.

6. The incisions are sewn closed.

Duration: 4 hours.

What to expect when it's over:

Pain medication often is given through the catheter that is already in place for anesthesia.

Patients are generally in the hospital about 5 to 7 days.

There may be swelling in the leg, which is temporary, but can last for several days or weeks.

Walking is gradually resumed, often with the help of a physical therapist. Continued physical therapy may be necessary, depending on how mobile the patient was before the surgery.

In most cases, walking improves and symptoms, such as pain and foot ulcers, go away.

PHLEBECTOMY/VARICOSE VEIN REMOVAL

Valves in the surface veins of the legs may become defective and cause the blood passing through them to pool. The resulting swollen and distorted veins and their branches are removed or divided and tied off.

Part of the body operated on:
The thigh and/or the calf.

Reasons for having the operation:
To improve circulation of the blood by removing diseased veins that hurt circulation, and by redirecting blood into healthy veins.
To avoid complications that include: pain, swelling, skin problems such as inflammation and discoloration, clot formation in the vein, bleeding, ulcers.

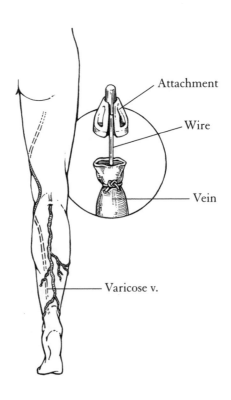

Attachment

Wire

Vein

Varicose v.

What could happen if you don't have the operation:
Increase in the size and distribution of the varicose veins.
Progressive leg swelling and pain.
Skin damage leading to dermatitis, inflammation, and ulceration.
Areas of rupture with bleeding.
Clot formation (phlebitis).

Factors that increase your risk of complications:
Cancer.
Diabetes.
Heart disease.
Kidney, lung, or liver disorders.
Obesity.
Prior episodes of phlebitis.
Prior leg surgery.
Scarring or inflammation.

Possible complications during and after surgery:
Complications are uncommon, but could include:

Bleeding, infection, wound separation.
Deep vein phlebitis or blood clots in the lung known as pulmonary emboli (rarely).
Stretched or cut skin nerves leading to temporary, but sometimes prolonged or permanent, changes in sensation, like numbness, "pins and needles," touch sensitivity, or pain.

Tests you may have to undergo:
Blood tests (count, chemistry, and clotting).
Chest X ray.
EKG.
Leg ultrasound (to make sure the deep veins in the muscles are healthy and to identify which surface veins or vein segments are diseased and need to be removed).
Urinalysis.

Basic steps of the operation:
1. Varicose veins are marked on the skin with the patient in a standing position.

2. General or spinal anesthesia is administered. The leg is cleansed, prepped, and draped.
3. A half-inch cut is made above or beside the ankle to locate the lower end of either the vein that runs along the entire inner leg (great saphenous vein) or the vein that extends from the ankle to the back of the knee (lesser saphenous vein).
4. A cable is introduced and passed upwards to the other end of the vein (either the groin or knee). Another cut is made where the upper end is located and the branches of the vein are divided and tied.
5. The end of the cut vein is secured to the cable and pulled down or up to remove (strip) its entire length. The branches that are disrupted by this maneuver will clot and stop bleeding without being separately tied.
6. Any other sites of varicosities that were identified are elevated through separate stab wounds or incisions of about one-quarter to one inch. They are either pulled out or divided and tied.
7. The wounds are closed with sutures or staples.

Duration: 3 hours.

What to expect when it's over:

When the patient wakes up, the leg aches, but it is not an intense or severe pain. Bandages cover the calf and thigh. They are slightly restrictive, but they do not impede walking.

Walking is encouraged and leg elevation is advised when not walking. Standing or sitting for more than a brief period should be avoided.

When the bandages are removed, there will be black-and-blue marks, particularly along the vein-stripping path. These will gradually fade and disappear over several weeks.

Bathing or showering is permitted 3 to 7 days after surgery; staples or sutures are removed in 1 to 2 weeks.

Normal sedentary activity is generally possible within 1 to several days, full unrestricted activity within 2 to 4 weeks.

Skin marks and scar lumpiness are initially prominent, but gradually fade and soften over several weeks to several months. The scars continue to evolve, usually becoming lighter and thinner, over several years. In some patients, scars may remain prominent or form keloids (dense wide scars).

Circulation of the blood in the leg is improved. Surface veins carry about 15 percent of the blood in the leg. When they are diseased, they hurt circulation because of stagnating or reversed flow. When they are removed, blood is forced into healthy veins deep in the muscles.

Surface veins that have been removed or tied off will not be available for bypass procedures, if needed at a later date. However, if a vein has become diseased it could not be used in any case.

Often small residual varicose veins remain since surgical removal of all abnormal vein segments is rarely possible. These may be treated by injection (sclerotherapy).

Recurrence of varicose veins is not uncommon. Often these are few and scattered and can either be left alone, injected, or removed in a minor office procedure under local anesthesia. Preventive measures include wearing elastic support stockings, regular walking, standing as little as possible, and sitting with the feet elevated.

Resources

There are hundreds of organizations devoted to specific diseases or medical problems. Your physician should be able to provide contact information for those relevant to your condition. I have listed surgical and health-care consumer contact information, organizations, books, and Web sites to help you find second opinions or do other research.

COLUMBIA PRESBYTERIAN CENTER NEW YORK-PRESBYTERIAN HOSPITAL SURGEONS' CONTACT INFORMATION

Columbia Presbyterian Center Physician Referral Service
800-277-2762

Amory, Spencer
PHONE: 212-932-5221
FAX: 212-932-5425
E-MAIL: SEA1@columbia.edu
Hemorrhoidectomy
Gallbladder Removal
Peptic Ulcer Surgery

Ascherman, Jeffrey
PHONE: 212-305-9612

FAX: 212-305-9626
E-MAIL: JAA2@columbia.edu
Breast Reconstruction
Carpal Tunnel Syndrome Repair
Cleft Lip Repair
Ganglion Cyst Removal

Benson, Mitchell C.
PHONE: 212-305-5201
FAX: 212-305-6813

E-MAIL: MCB2@columbia.edu
Prostatectomy

Benvenisty, Alan
PHONE: 212-305-8055
FAX: 212-305-4140
E-MAIL: AIB3@columbia.edu
Lower Extremity Arterial Bypass

Bessler, Marc
PHONE: 212-305-9506
FAX: 212-305-5992
E-MAIL: mb28@columbia.edu
Esophogeal Surgery
Gastric Bypass

Bigliani, Louis
PHONE: 212-305-5564
FAX: 212-305-4040
E-MAIL: lub1@columbia.edu
Rotator Cuff Repair

Chabot, John
PHONE: 212-305-9468
FAX: 212-305-5992
E-MAIL: JAC@columbia.edu
Pancreatectomy

Chaglassian, Ted
PHONE: 212-305-5499
FAX: 212-305-5233
Melanoma/Skin Lesion Removal

Cotliar, Arthur
PHONE: 212-305-2241
FAX: 212-305-3266
E-MAIL: Acotliar@aol.com
Cataract Removal

Ditkoff, BethAnn
PHONE: 212-305-1050
FAX: 212-305-1060
Mastectomy/Breast Lumpectomy

Edwards, Niloo
PHONE: 212-305-9242
FAX: 212-305-2439
E-MAIL: NME3@columbia.edu
Heart Transplantation

Huang, Emina Hui-na
PHONE: 212-305-2676
FAX: 212-305-5992
Colorectal Resection

Geller, Peter
PHONE: 212-305-6657
FAX: 212-305-2074
E-MAIL: plg@columbia.edu
Appendectomy
Hernia Repair

Ginsburg, Mark
PHONE: 212-305-3408
FAX: 212-305-3474
E-MAIL: meg18@columbia.edu
Lung Transplantation/Lung Removal

Gorenstein, Lyall
PHONE: 212-305-3408
FAX: 212-305-3474
E-MAIL: lag17@columbia.edu
Lung Transplantation/Lung Removal

Hardy, Mark
PHONE: 212-305-5502
FAX: 212-305-4061

E-MAIL: MAHL@columbia.edu
Kidney Transplant

Kenneth A. Forde
PHONE: 212-305-2735
FAX: 212-305-3236
E-MAIL: kaf2@columbia.edu
Colorectal Resection

Kiernan, Howard
PHONE: 212-305-5241
FAX: 212-305-1577
E-MAIL: kiernan@ortho1.cpmc.
columbia.edu
Arthroscopy

Levine, Richard
PHONE: 212-305-5300
FAX: 212-305-1142
E-MAIL: leviner@hermes.cpmc.
columbia.edu
Laparoscopy

Levine, William
PHONE: 305-0762
FAX: 305-4040
E-MAIL: wn19001@ortho1.
cpmc.columbia.edu
Arthroplasty (Knee Replacement)

LoGerfo, Paul
PHONE: 212-305-0444
FAX: 212-305-0445
E-MAIL: md180@columbia.edu
Parathyroidectomy
Thyroidectomy

Matera, Cristina
PHONE: 212-639-9122

FAX: 212-639-9413
Tubal Ligation

Nowygrod, Roman
PHONE: 212-305-5374
FAX: 212-305-1563
Varicose Vein Removal

Oz, Mehmet
PHONE: 212-305-4434
FAX: 212-305-2439
E-MAIL: mco2@columbia.edu
Heart Valve Replacement and
Repair/Coronary Artery Bypass

Parks, Michael
PHONE: 212-305-0403
FAX: 212-305-4024
E-MAIL: mlp48@columbia.edu
Hip Replacement

Rabbani, LeRoy
PHONE: 212-305-1581
FAX: 212-305-3679
Angioplasty

Rubin, David
PHONE: 914-428-3888
FAX: 914-686-5366
Radiofrequency Ablation

Schnabel, Freya
PHONE: 212-305-1534
FAX: 212-305-1522
Breast Lumpectomy

Smith, Daniel H.
PHONE: 212-305-3410

FAX: 212-305-3412
Hysterectomy

Solomon, Robert
PHONE: 212-305-4118
FAX: 212-305-2026
Cerebral Aneurysm Repair

Spotnitz, Henry
PHONE: 212-305-6191
FAX: 212-305-9724
E-MAIL: hms2@columbia.edu
Pacemaker Insertion

Thomashow, Byron
PHONE: 212-305-5261
FAX: 212-305-1386
Bronchoscopy

Todd, George
PHONE: 212-305-5505
FAX: 212-305-4199
*Abdominal Aortic Aneurysm
Repair/Carotid Artery
Endarterectomy*

Weidenbaum, Mark
PHONE: 212-305-3962
FAX: 212-305-4024
E-MAIL: weidenb@orthol.
cpmc.columbia.edu
*Scoliosis Surgery
Discectomy/Lumbar Disk
Surgery*

ORGANIZATIONS

National Insurance Consumer Helpline
American Council of Life Insurance
Health Insurance Association of America
1001 Pennsylvania Avenue, NW
Washington, DC 20004
800-942-4242

Provides general information on how to choose an agent or broker and insurance company.

Medic Alert Foundation International
2323 N. Colorado Avenue
Turlock, CA 95380
900-432-5378

Provides information on how to register with Medic Alert to obtain an emergency identification bracelet.

Inspector General's Hotline
U.S. Department of Health and Human Services
P.O. Box 17303
Baltimore, MD 21203
800-368-5779

Handles complaints relating to overcharges and possible fraud in Medicare and Medicaid programs.

Medicare Information Hotline
U.S. Department of Health and Human Services
Washington, DC 20201
800-888-1770 (recorded message)
800-888-1998 (requests for information, written material)

Provides general information on the Medicare program and responds to questions about Medicare coverage.

Medicare Medigap Insurance Fraud Line
U.S. Department of Health and Human Services
Washington, DC 20201
800-638-6833

Provides information on supplemental Medicare or Medigap policies.

BOOKS

American Medical Association Family Medical Guide, edited by Charles B. Clayman, Random House, 1994.
The Best Doctors in America, by Steven Naifeh and Gregory White Smith, Woodward/White, Inc., 1997 (3rd Edition).
The Columbia University College of Physicians and Surgeons Complete Home Medical Guide, edited by Genell J. Subak-Sharpe and Donald F. Tapley, Crown Books, 1995.
Healing from the Heart: A Leading Heart Surgeon Explores the Power of Complementary Medicine, by Mehmet Oz, Dutton, 1998.
How to Find the Best Doctors: New York Metro Area, by John J. Connolly, Castle Connolly Medical, Ltd., 1998.
The Physicians' Desk Reference Family Guide Encyclopedia of Medical Care, Three Rivers Press, 1997.

The Physicians' Desk Reference Pocket Guide to Prescription Drugs,
Three Rivers Press, 1999.

WEB SITES

American Academy of Ophthalmology
http://www.eyenet.org

American Academy of Orthopedic Surgeons
http://www.aaos.org

American Association of Neurological Surgeons
http://www.neurosurgery.org

American College of Obstetricians and Gynecologists
http://www.acog.org

American College of Surgeons
http://www.facs.org

American Society of Colon and Rectal Surgeons
http://www.fascrs.org

American Society of Transplant Surgeons
http://www.asts.org

American Trauma Society
http://www.amtrauma.org

American Urological Association
http://www.auanet.org

Columbia Presbyterian Center
http://www.cpmcnet.columbia.edu

Columbia Presbyterian Department of Surgery
http://www.columbiasurgery.org

New York-Presbyterian Hospital
http://www.nyp.org

Royal College of Surgeons of England
http://www.rcseng.ac.uk

Society of American Gastrointestinal Endoscopic Surgeons
http://www.sages.org

Society of Critical Care Medicine
http://www.sccm.org

Society of Thoracic Surgeons
http://www.sts.org

Spine Surgery
http://www.spine-surgery.com

Vascular Surgery Societies
http://www.vascsurg.org

WebMD
http://www.webmd.com

APPENDIX B

Sample Living Will

Note: The following form is for information
purposes only. It is not a valid form.

DIRECTIVE MADE this ___ day of _____, 2000, to my
physicians, my attorneys, my clergyman, my family or others responsible for my health, welfare, or affairs.
BE IT KNOWN that I, _____, of the
State of _____, being an adult of sound mind, will-
fully and voluntarily make this statement as a directive to be followed if I am in a terminal condition and become unable to
participate in decisions regarding my health care. I understand that
my health-care providers are legally bound to act consistently with
my wishes, within the limits of responsible medical practice and
other applicable law. I also understand that I have the right to make
medical and health-care decisions for myself as long as I am able to
do so and to revoke this declaration at any time.

DURABLE POWER OF ATTORNEY

I understand that my wishes expressed in the following cases may
not cover all possible aspects of my care if I become incompetent. I
also may be undecided about whether I want a particular treatment
or not. Consequently, there may be a need for someone to accept or
refuse medical intervention for me in consultation with my physicians. I authorize:

Either/or
1) Name _____ Phone _____
Address _____ Relationship _____
2) Name _____ Phone _____
Address _____ Relationship _____
as my proxy(s) to make the decision for me whenever my wishes expressed in this document are insufficient or undecided.
Should there be any disagreement between the wishes I have indicated in this document and the decisions favored by my above proxy(s) to have authority over any medical directive/ I wish my medical directive to have authority over my proxy(s). (Please delete as necessary.)
Should there be any disagreement between the wishes of my proxies,
Name _____ Phone _____
Address _____ Relationship _____

shall have final authority.

Signed in the presence of:

_____   _____
Witness   Address

_____   _____
Witness   Address

Sample Health-Care Proxy

Note: The following form is for information purposes only. It is not a valid form.

1. I, _____, hereby appoint _____ _____ as my health-care agent, to make any and all health-care decisions for me, except to the extent that I state otherwise. This proxy shall take effect when and if I become unable to make by own health-care decisions.

2. Optional instructions: I direct my proxy to make health-care decisions in accord with my wishes and limitations as stated below, or as he or she otherwise knows. (Unless your agent knows your wishes about artificial nutrition and hydration [feeding tubes], your agent will not be allowed to make decisions about artificial nutrition and hydration.)

3. Name of substitute or fill-in proxy if the person I appoint above is unable, unwilling, or unavailable to act as my health-care agent: _____.

4. Unless I revoke it, this proxy shall remain in effect indefinitely, or until the date or conditions stated below. The proxy shall expire (specific date or conditions, if desired): _____
_____

5. Signature _____
   Address _____
   Date _____

6. Statement by Witnesses (must be 18 or older). I declare that the person who signed this document is personally known to me and appears to be of sound mind and acting of his or her own free will. He or she signed (or asked another to sign for him or her) this document in my presence.

Witness 1 _____
Address _____
Witness 2 _____
Address _____

This form will become part of your hospital records.

Sample Consent Form

Note: The following form is for information purposes only. It is not a valid form.

Informed consent for surgical operation, diagnostic and other therapeutic procedures.

I give permission for the surgical operation, diagnostic or therapeutic procedures listed below and/or blood transfusions upon myself or the patient named above.

List of Procedures: _____
_____
_____
_____

I have been advised that the procedures will be performed by Dr. _____ and his assistants. I request and consent to these procedures and other procedures which are deemed advisable by my physicians during the course of treatment. Any organs or tissues which are surgically removed may be examined and retained by the hospital for medical, scientific, or educational purposes and may be disposed of according to customary practices.

Restrictions: _____
_____
(State restrictions or None)

The nature and purpose of the procedures, the expected discomforts, risks, complications, and benefits and the alternative treatments, if any, have been fully explained to me. I acknowledge that no guarantees or assurances have been made to me concerning the results intended from the procedures. I have been given the opportunity to ask questions and all my questions have been answered fully and satisfactorily by:

Dr.: _____
Signature

Signed: _____ (Patient)
Date: _____

When a patient is a minor or incompetent to give consent:

Signed: _____
Signature of person authorized
to consent for patient

Relationship to patient: _____

A Patient's Bill of Rights

A Patient's Bill of Rights was first adopted by the American Hospital Association in 1973.
This revision was approved by the AHA Board of Trustees on October 21, 1992.

These rights can be exercised on the patient's behalf by a designated surrogate or proxy decision maker if the patient lacks decision-making capacity, is legally incompetent, or is a minor.

1. The patient has the right to considerate and respectful care.

2. The patient has the right to and is encouraged to obtain from physicians and other direct caregivers relevant, current, and understandable information concerning diagnosis, treatment, and prognosis.

   Except in emergencies when the patient lacks decision-making capacity and the need for treatment is urgent, the patient is entitled to the opportunity to discuss and request information related to the specific procedures and/or treatments, the risks involved, the possible length of recuperation, and the medically reasonable alternatives and their accompanying risks and benefits.

Patients have the right to know the identity of physicians, nurses, and others involved in their care, as well as when those involved are students, residents, or other trainees. The patient also has the right to know the immediate and long-term financial implications of treatment choices, insofar as they are known.

3. The patient has the right to make decisions about the plan of care prior to and during the course of treatment and to refuse a recommended treatment or plan of care to the extent permitted by law and hospital policy and to be informed of the medical consequences of this action. In case of such refusal, the patient is entitled to other appropriate care and services that the hospital provides or transfer to another hospital. The hospital should notify patients of any policy that might affect patient choice within the institution.

4. The patient has the right to have an advance directive (such as a living will, health-care proxy, or durable power of attorney for health care) concerning treatment or designating a surrogate decision maker with the expectation that the hospital will honor the intent of that directive to the extent permitted by law and hospital policy. Health-care institutions must advise patients of their rights under state law and hospital policy to make informed medical choices, ask if the patient has an advance directive, and include that information in patient records. The patient has the right to timely information about hospital policy that may limit its ability to implement fully a legally valid advance directive.

5. The patient has the right to every consideration of privacy. Case discussion, consultation, examination, and treatment should be conducted so as to protect each patient's privacy.

6. The patient has the right to expect that all communications and records pertaining to his/her care will be treated as confidential by the hospital, except in cases such as suspected abuse and public health hazards when reporting is permitted or required by law. The patient has the right to expect that the hospital will emphasize the confidentiality of this information when it re-

leases it to any other parties entitled to review information in these records.

7. The patient has the right to review the records pertaining to his/her medical care and to have the information explained or interpreted as necessary, except when restricted by law.

8. The patient has the right to expect that, within its capacity and policies, a hospital will make a reasonable response to the request of a patient for appropriate and medically indicated care and services. The hospital must provide evaluation, service, and/or referral as indicated by the urgency of the case. When medically appropriate and legally permissible, or when a patient has so requested, a patient may be transferred to another facility. The institution to which the patient is to be transferred must first have accepted the patient for transfer. The patient must also have the benefit of complete information and explanation concerning the need for, risks, benefits, and alternatives to such a transfer.

9. The patient has the right to ask and be informed of the existence of business relationships among the hospital, educational institutions, other health-care providers, or payers that may influence the patient's treatment and care.

10. The patient has the right to consent to or decline to participate in proposed research studies or human experimentation affecting care and treatment or requiring direct patient involvement, and to have those studies fully explained prior to consent. A patient who declines to participate in research or experimentation is entitled to the most effective care that the hospital can otherwise provide.

11. The patient has the right to expect reasonable continuity of care when appropriate and to be informed by physicians and other caregivers of available and realistic patient-care options when hospital care is no longer appropriate.

12. The patient has the right to be informed of hospital policies and practices that relate to patient care, treatment, and responsibilities. The patient has the right to be informed of available re-

sources for resolving disputes, grievances, and conflicts, such as ethics committees, patient representatives, or other mechanisms available in the institution. The patient has the right to be informed of the hospital's charges for services and available payment methods.

APPENDIX F

Sample Appointment Schedule

APPOINTMENT SCHEDULE

Date	Reason for visit	Your questions	Doctor's answers and instructions

Sample Appointment Schedule

Date	Reason for visit	Your questions	Doctor's answers and instructions

Checklist of Questions

CHECKLIST OF QUESTIONS FOR YOUR PRIMARY SURGEON:

- What part of my body is diseased or injured?

- What does it do when it's functioning normally?

- What's it doing in my case?

- How does this affect me?

- What are my chances of ridding myself of the problem through surgery?

- What is the chance that specific symptoms will improve?

- How much improvement can I expect in how I feel or in my life expectancy?

- What is the chance the symptoms or disease will recur?

- Where do these figures come from and how valid are they?

- If I don't have this operation, what might I expect?

- How many of these procedures have you done?

- What are your clinical outcomes for this procedure?

If you're considering a second opinion, ask yourself:

- How serious is my condition?

- Should I be getting independent verification about the information I've heard?

- Is there any chance that I could be following a course that's not the best?

- How big an impact will the decision I'm making now have on my life?

- How do I feel about my doctor and my interaction with him?

- Do I have any doubts about anything I've heard?

- What do I have to lose if I take my records across town and say to another doctor, "What do you think?"

APPENDIX H

Post-Operative Instruction Form

YOUR DOCTOR'S POST-OPERATIVE INSTRUCTIONS:

1. _____

2. _____

3. _____

4. _____

5. _____

6. _____

7. _____

8. _____

9. _____

10. _____

APPENDIX I

Prescription Timetable Form

YOUR PRESCRIPTION TIMETABLE

Date	Medication	Frequency/ dose	Taken	Refills

Prescription Timetable Form

Date	Medication	Frequency/ dose	Taken	Refills

Index